ABSOLUTE
Perfection!

by the editors of

oxygen

Published by Robert Kennedy Publishing
5775 McLaughlin Road
Mississauga ON
L5R 3P7
Canada

Designed and edited by Wendy Morley
Library and Archives Canada Cataloguing in Publication

Absolute perfection : your complete program for a slim, lean waistline (an amazing body, too!) / by the editors of Oxygen magazine.

ISBN-13: 978-1-55210-037-0
ISBN-10: 1-55210-037-5

1. Abdominal exercises. 2. Exercise for women.

GV482.A38 2006   613.7'1886082
C2006-906748-1

10 9 8 7 6 5 4 3 2 1

Distributed by NBN Books
Head Office
4501 Forbes Blvd.
Suite 200
Lanham, MD 20706

Distribution Center
15200 NBN Way
Blue Ridge Summit, PA 17214

Printed in Canada

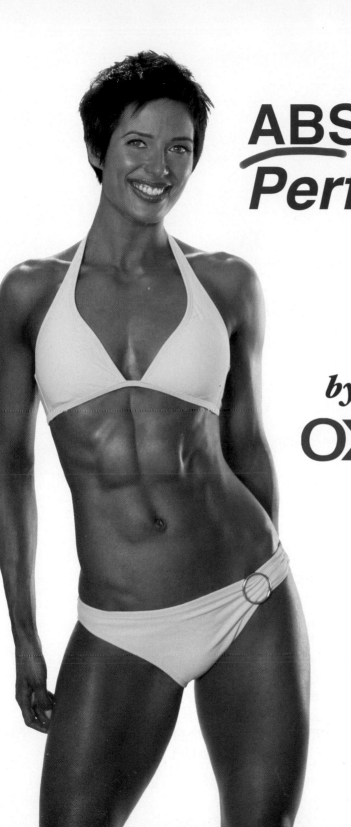

ABSOLUTE
Perfection!

by the editors of
oxygen

Table of Contents

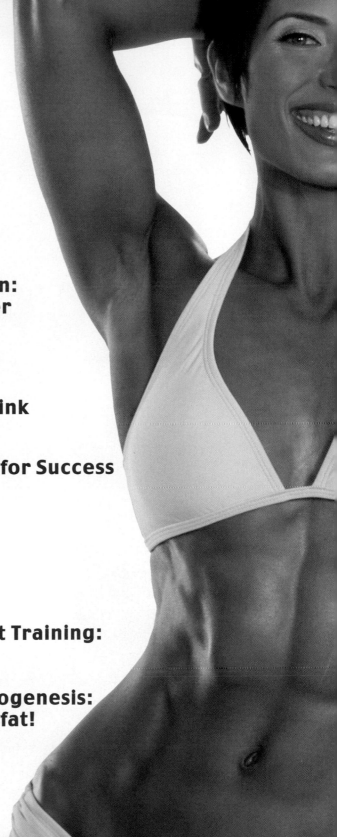

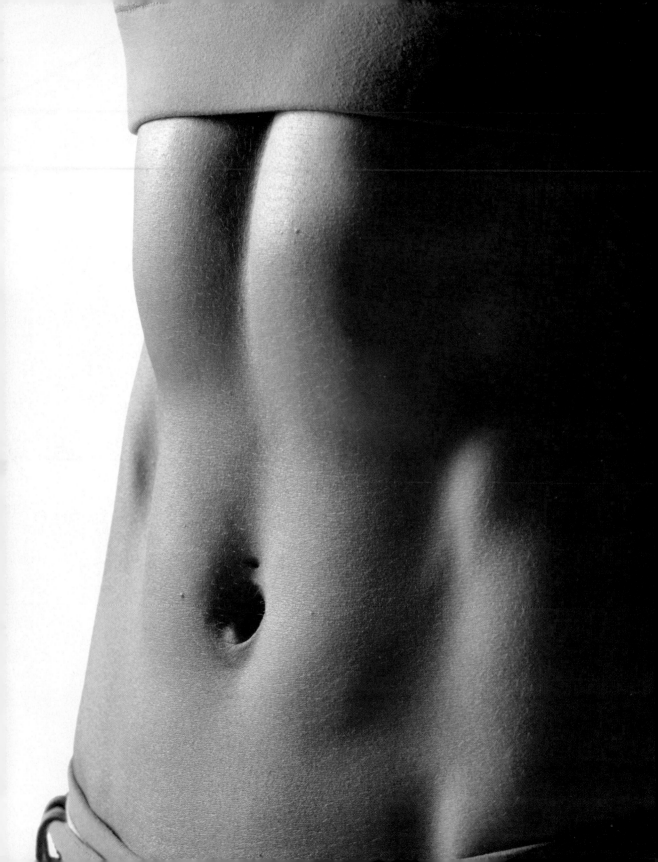

Foreword by Robert Kennedy

The Promise of Amazing Abdominals

Nothing screams fit and sexy like a slim, tight waistline with a flat belly. And this book is devoted to helping you achieve just that.

But this achievement takes more than a few crunches. You need a program that will do more than just strengthen your abdominal muscles. What good are strong abdominals that lie hidden behind pounds of jiggly fat? You need a program that leans you out while toning and strengthening your whole body. As the focal point of that fabulous body you will also create a phenomenal midsection. What more could you want?

Make the decision. Make it right now. Decide that, using the tools we provide, you are going to forge yourself a stunning body. Do you have a full-length mirror? If so, go to it right this second. Bring this book along with you. If you don't have a full-length mirror, go to the largest mirror you have. Now take off your clothes. All of them. Take a good, long, hard look at yourself Do you like what you see? If so, great. Keep doing what you're doing. The rest of you, look through that fat. See past your thick waistline to the trim, neat little waist hidden inside. Visualize your body exactly as you want it to be. If you follow this program, that body will be yours.

Now put your clothes back on. Say out loud, "Yes! I want a waistline that models would envy! I can't wait to get going on this program and show off my new body. I *will* follow the advice in this book. I *will* exercise hard. I *will* be consistent. I *will* follow a clean diet. I will start today. I will start this very minute! While I know the results won't come overnight, I know they will come if I persevere. I cannot fail. I will succeed."

And believe it. You will succeed. I know you will.

Chapter 1
Motivation
harnessing your inner power

To excel in any endeavor you must be hungry – hungry for success. It starts with a dream, but somehow you must be inspired, or you will never be able to reach your goal. We often read about athletes overcoming physical disabilities. Lance Armstrong survived testicular cancer and won the Tour de France seven times. Marla Runyan ran in the 1500 meters at the 2000 Olympics while legally blind. Out of these challenges athletes develop a fierce, burning desire to succeed. They need

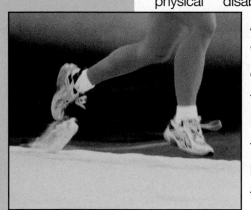

to prove to themselves that they can achieve their goals. Through these kinds of examples we can begin to understand that *desire* is sometimes more important than talent, or even a healthy body.

Without a true commitment to be the best you can be, you will never be able to push yourself to do what has to be done. It will be too easy to skip a workout now and then. A coach, spouse or friend can give you support and guidance, but *you* have to supply the rest. Only you can push yourself when you're tired, or make yourself work out when distractions get in the way.

The drive must come from within, whatever you are trying to succeed at. The good news is that building and maintaining a high level of self-motivation is a skill anyone can acquire. Motivation is one of the most powerful sources of energy available to any successful person. From internal motivation you gain the willingness to persevere with your training, to endure discomfort and stress and to make sacrifices with your time and energy as you move closer towards realizing your goal.

Profile of the Highly Motivated Person

What are the key characteristics of highly successful people? The characteristics that make an athlete a champion, that make an actor a movie star, or simply make a woman able to finally get rid of her belly fat can be attained and developed by anyone who wants to excel.

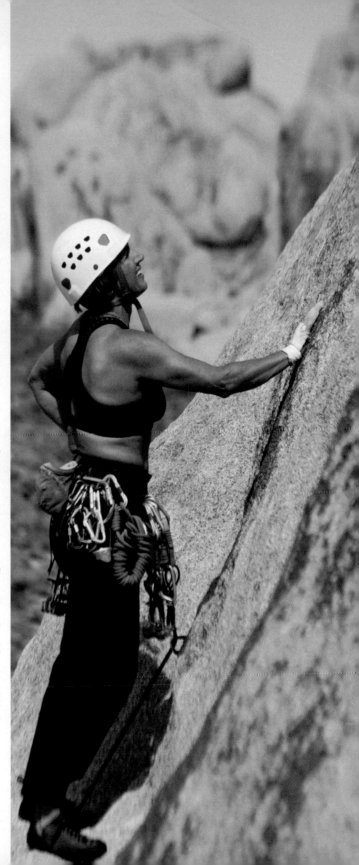

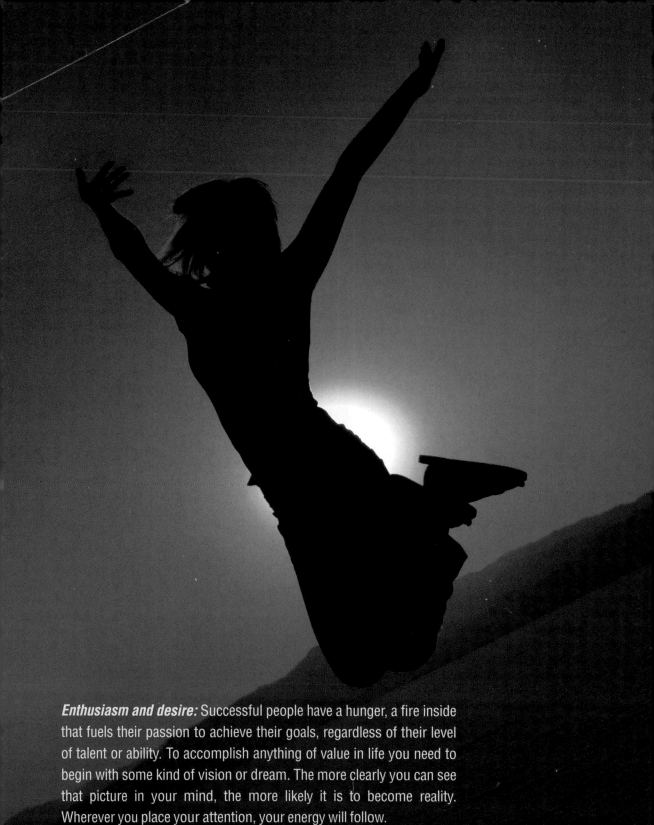

Enthusiasm and desire: Successful people have a hunger, a fire inside that fuels their passion to achieve their goals, regardless of their level of talent or ability. To accomplish anything of value in life you need to begin with some kind of vision or dream. The more clearly you can see that picture in your mind, the more likely it is to become reality. Wherever you place your attention, your energy will follow.

Self-direction

You cannot be successful unless you are doing this for yourself. Losing weight for a reunion? It will reappear when it's over. Losing weight to make your husband happy? You'll be sneaking chocolates when he's not looking. Direction and drive need to come from within. You must choose your own goals because they lead you to the person you want to be.

Commitment to excellence

How good do you want to be? To excel at anything you must decide to make it a priority in your life. Make an honest effort every day to be the best at what you do. At some point you must say to yourself, 'I truly want this to work.' You must live this commitment. Regularly stretch what you perceive to be your current limits.

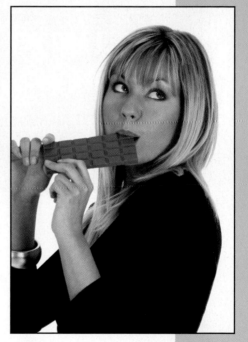

Discipline, consistency, organization

Winning people know how to self-energize and work hard on a daily basis. If you truly want your body to look amazing; if you truly want to have a slim, firm waistline, you must maintain consistency. Regardless of personal problems, fatigue, or difficult circumstances, you must find a way to generate enough excitement and energy to do your best. If you always keep the end result in sight, this becomes much easier.

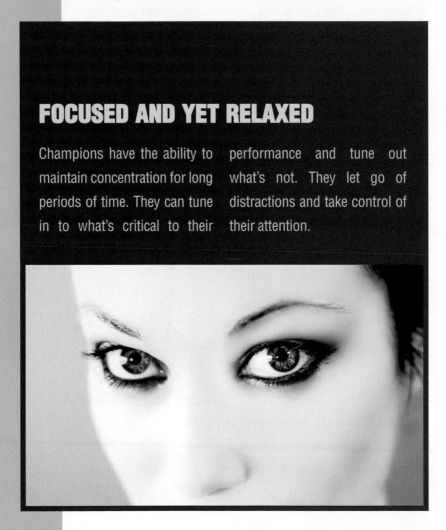

FOCUSED AND YET RELAXED

Champions have the ability to maintain concentration for long periods of time. They can tune in to what's critical to their performance and tune out what's not. They let go of distractions and take control of their attention.

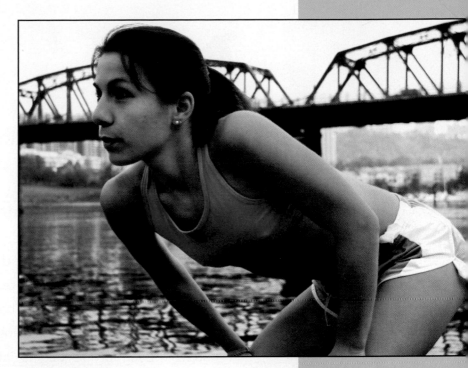

Ability to handle adversity

Any successful person simply deals with difficult situations. Adversity builds character. When a successful woman knows the odds are against her she embraces the chance to explore the outer limits of her potential. Rather than avoiding pressure she feels challenged by it. Champions are calm and relaxed under fire. Setbacks become an opportunity for learning; they open the way for deep personal growth.

Guidelines for Building Motivation
and
Maximizing Your Potential

The people who develop these qualities and practice these skills regularly have the best chance of excelling in any endeavor. Each of us begins at a different starting point, physically and mentally. We all have strengths we can build upon. Now that you have an idea of the constellation of traits successful people possess, how do you begin to build them into your life? How do you turn these qualities into useful behaviors that will make a difference in the way you live every day? Here are some suggestions that may help you in your quest for better health and fitness.

Generate a positive outlook

Direct your focus to what is possible; to what can happen; towards success. Rather than complaining about the weather or thinking about how you'd rather be watching your favorite TV show, picture yourself buying a bikini for the first time in however many years. **You have control** over your thoughts, your emotions, and how you perceive each situation. **You choose** what you believe about yourself. Positive energy makes success possible.

Practice being focused and yet relaxed

Develop the ability to maintain concentration for longer periods of time. Tune in to what's critical to your goal and tune out what's not. You can easily let go of distractions and take control of your attention. As you focus more on the task at hand there will be less room for negative thoughts to enter your mind.

> Positive energy makes peak performance possible.

Build a balanced lifestyle

Create a broad-based lifestyle with a variety of interests. Strive for a balance between work and fun, social time, personal quiet time and time to be creative. Develop patterns of healthy behavior. Eat regularly, get a consistent amount of sleep each night. If possible, reduce your workload at times and allow time to relax and reflect between activities. Develop a social support network of close friends and family who have many different interests. Sure, it's great to have people around with the same interests and goals as you have, but opening your mind and life up to new possibilities can make success easier to find. Learn to communicate openly; resolve personal conflicts as they occur, so they don't build to a crisis and threaten your plans.

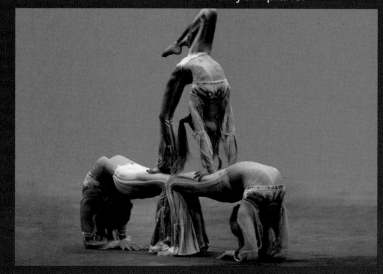

Vary your workouts

Train at a new, scenic place at least once a week. This doesn't have to be an actual gym – train outside for a change. You'll get a tremendous psychological boost and will likely improve your fitness level. Put a new spark in your training schedule by trying interval work, tempo work (fast 20- to 30-minute training sessions) and varying your speed. If your workouts are the same, day after day or week after week, not only will they not be as effective for you, you will get bored. Soon you'll be finding excuses not to do them.

Enjoy your training

Make a deliberate effort each day to create enjoyment in your training. Renew your enthusiasm and excitement. Don't try to force your physical improvement. Let your breakthrough occur naturally, at its own pace, when the internal conditions are ideal. Use setbacks as learning opportunities. Try to draw out constructive lessons from every workout and then move on. Look for advantages in every situation, even if the conditions are less than ideal.

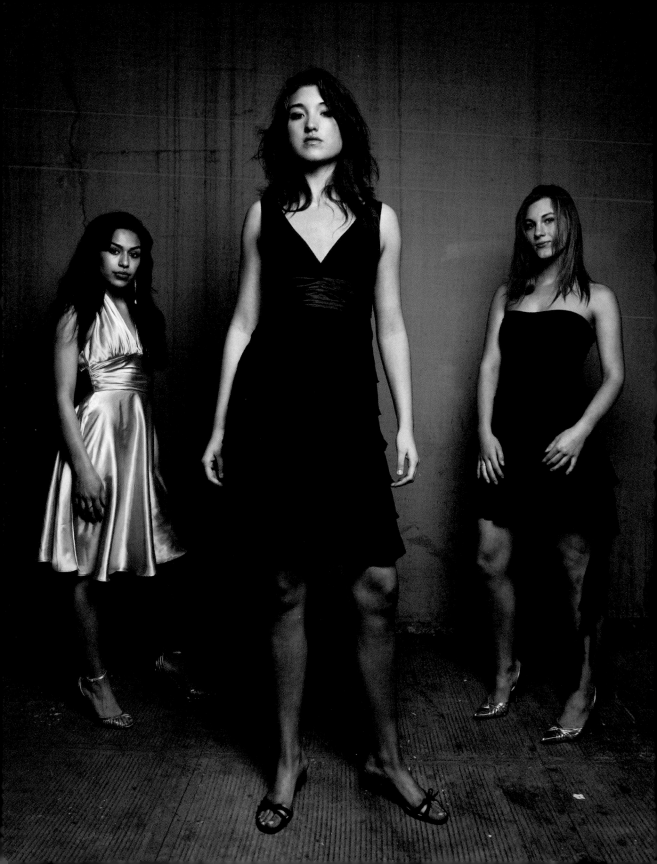

Chapter 2

What "Type" Are You?

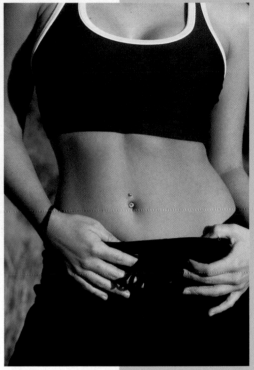

W e've all heard the phrase "oh, she's naturally big boned" or "he was always muscular." Most people have a certain genetic body type that can be easily identified with just a quick glance. Physiologists use the term *somatotype* to describe an individual's natural body shape. Somatotypes take into account numerous physical variables including a person's body fat, bone structure and muscularity.

There are three primary categories of somatotypes – mesomorph, endomorph and ectomorph. In general terms, mesomorphs are naturally muscular; endomorphs tend to accumulate fat very easily; ectomorphs are the "skinny" types who have low body-fat levels and not much muscle mass. While a few people seem almost a stereotype of one category, most have characteristics of two or more.

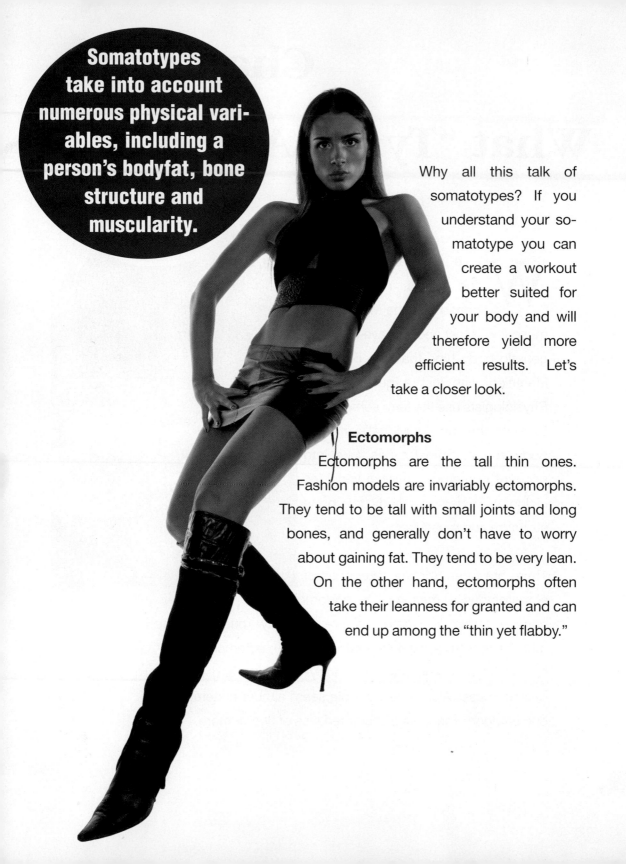

Why all this talk of somatotypes? If you understand your somatotype you can create a workout better suited for your body and will therefore yield more efficient results. Let's take a closer look.

Ectomorphs

Ectomorphs are the tall thin ones. Fashion models are invariably ectomorphs. They tend to be tall with small joints and long bones, and generally don't have to worry about gaining fat. They tend to be very lean. On the other hand, ectomorphs often take their leanness for granted and can end up among the "thin yet flabby."

Mesomorph

Mesomorphs look, and often are, athletic. Male mesomorphs tend to be quite muscular, females are often described as having an hourglass figure. Of course, many female mesomorphs are also athletic. Demi Moore is a mesomorph, as was Jayne Mansfield.

Mesomorphs are naturally strong and usually do well at such sports as sprinting. You won't see a mesomorph winning a marathon. Pure mesomorphs stay lean fairly easily because of their high muscle ratios, but many are only an ice-cream scoop away from being considered fat. As they tend not to be especially tall, it doesn't take many extra pounds to make them appear overweight.

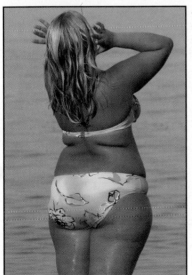

Endomorphs

For an image of an endomorph think of Ricky Lake, Roseanne Barr or Rosie O'Donnell. Politely speaking, endomorphs have a soft body with underdeveloped muscles. Endomorphs usually have a slow metabolism and gain fat very easily. Remember the chubby kid in grade four who every-one picked on? That's an endomorph. With large abdomen, long trunk and short legs, endomorphs make poor athletes. They wage a constant battle to keep weight off.

What "type" of training routine?

Somatotyping can play a role in designing a training routine. Mesomorphs don't need to do anything radical. Moderation is the key. A mesomorph should do about three sessions each of weight training and cardio per week. Cardio and weights can be done in the same workout or you can split them up and do weights one day, cardio the next – whichever fits better into your routine.

Are you an...

Endomorph? It's best to focus your attention on getting rid of body fat. Endomorphs need to follow a diet low in fat and simple carbohydrates. And by diet, we mean eating plan, not temporary weight-loss fix. Foods like bacon, butter, high-fat cheese, creamy salad dressings, cookies, candies, soft drinks and chocolate must go! You need to concentrate on burning fat and building muscle (muscle boosts your metabolism, causing you to burn more fat all the time). A good endomorph program would have you training at least four days a week. You can do your weights and cardio together in one workout or you can split them up.

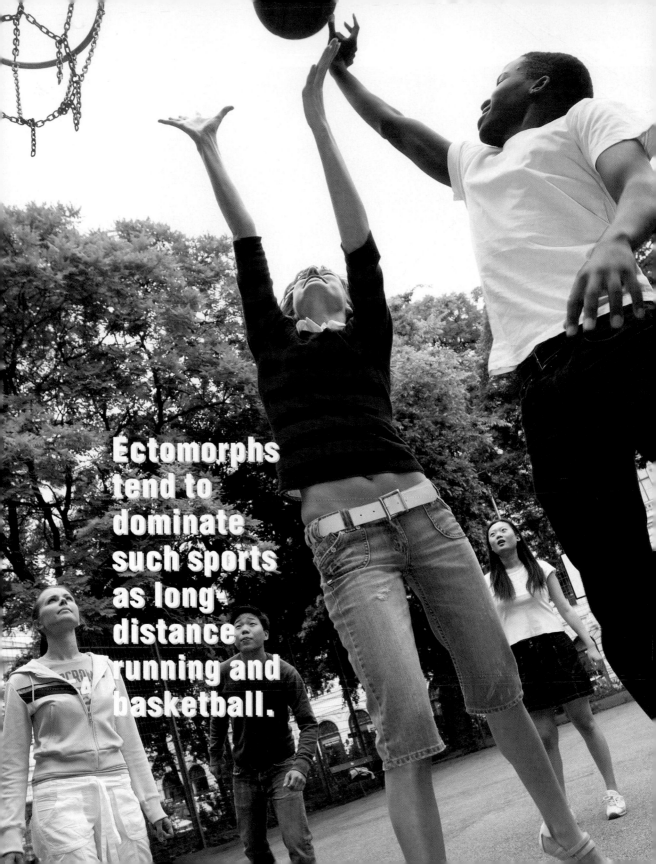

Ectomorphs tend to dominate such sports as long-distance running and basketball.

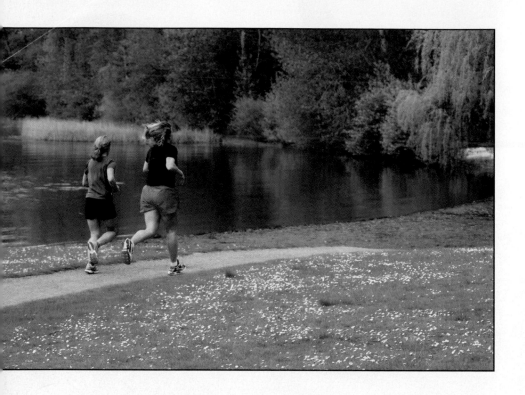

Endomorph Cardio Training

• For health reasons cardiovasular training is important for everyone. For weight-loss reasons it is especially important for you.

• You should do moderate-intenstiy cardio – jogging, walking briskly, bicycling, etc. – a minimum of three times a week for a minimum of 30 minutes each time. These are minimums! Getting up to six days a week and up to an hour and a half each time would be fine if you can fit it in your schedule. Just keep in mind that if you do that much you will have to mix days of lower intensity, like walking, with days of higher intensity, like jogging, to prevent injury and overtraining.

Endomorph Weight Training

• Train with weights at least two days a week, preferably three or four.

• Use your weight training to help burn fat – train with a weight that brings you to failure (meaning you can't do another) at 15 to 20 reps, for 3 sets. That means you lift the weight and bring it back down 15 to 20 times, rest for a minute, then repeat the sequence twice for a total of 3 sets.

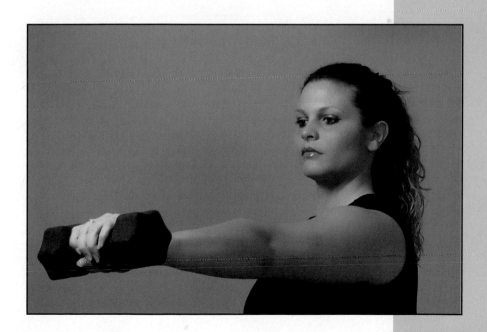

*Ab*solute Perfection

Ectomorphs have the opposite problem to endomorphs – they need to add some curves to their body. Even if the ectomorph is a little flabby, she should keep a fairly high (though healthy) caloric intake and do at least three days a week of weight training. For the ectomorph to get a firm yet curvy body, she will have to eat more frequently – four to six times per day. She should eat at least .7 grams of protein per pound of bodyweight.

Ectomorph Weight Training

• Ectomorphs should stick with basic compound exercises. That means exercises that involve more than one joint. For example, curling a dumbbell involves only the elbow joint – the elbow is the only joint that bends during a biceps curl. However, if you do a squat, you are bending the ankle, the knee, and the hip. Some other compound exercises include rows, shoulder presses, pushups, lat pulldowns, bench presses, and leg presses.

Train with weights three or four times a week, but stick to heavier weights that bring you to failure in 8 to 10 reps. You likely need to develop your strength.

Ectomorph Cardio Training

Everyone needs cardio for health, but keep yours at a lower intensity. Whereas the endomorph will want to bring her

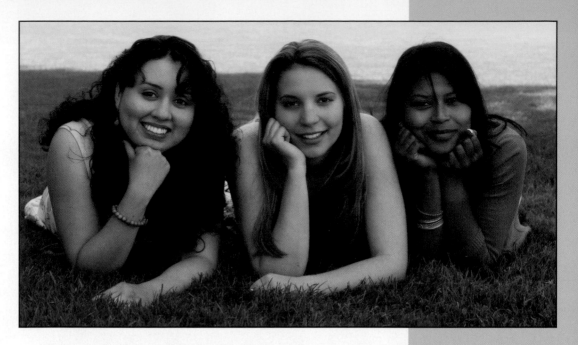

intensity level up considerably to burn more calories, you may want to stick to walking or fairly easy biking.

Mesomorphs will have to decide what they want their body to look like. They probably have the most flexible body type of all. Do you want to look long and lean like a fashion model? Well, you won't get quite that lanky, but you can certainly move in that direction by doing plenty of cardio, everything from low to high intensity, and by doing weights two or three times a week with low weights and high reps. Do you prefer the look of an athlete? Then you'll want to increase your weights and keep your reps lower – the 8 to 12 range.

In either case you will eat a well-balanced, clean diet, with four to six meals a day. If you want to be leaner you will simply eat less at each sitting.

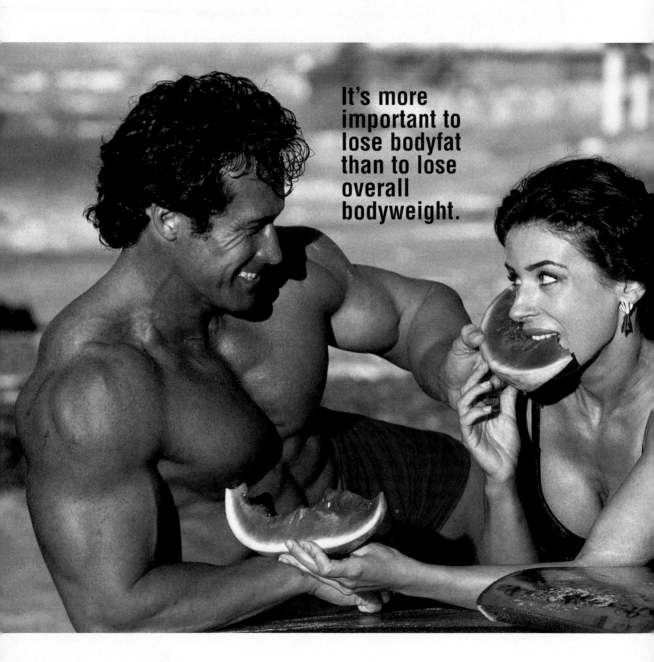

It's more important to lose bodyfat than to lose overall bodyweight.

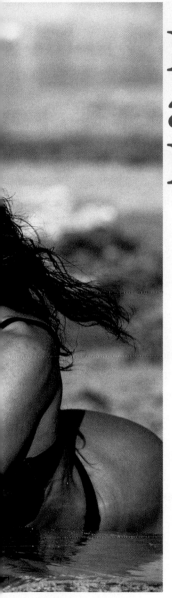

Chapter 3

Eat, Drink and Look Fabulous!

Y our nutritional needs vary depending upon your health and fitness goals. If your aim is to lose body fat and weight, you need to become familiar with the variables affecting the outcome of your efforts. Above all, you should realize it's more important to lose fat than to lose overall weight. Once you begin weight training you will develop muscle, which is much more dense than fat. So you can weigh more (and eat more!) but have a smaller, firmer body. Besides, you don't want a smaller, yet still flabby, body. It's best to reduce your intake of fatty foods and increase your level of physical activity, rather than just cutting calories.

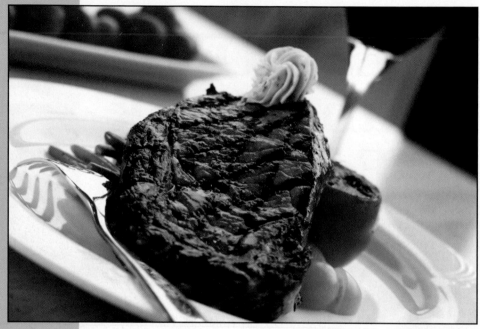

Calories

In simple terms a calorie, or kilocalorie (Kcal), is a measure of heat energy. Food calories are nutrients that supply energy to the body. It is essential to take in the minimal amount of calories per day. The caloric intake level appropriate for you depends on a number of factors, including your height, weight, gender and amount of physical activity. There are three types of nutrients that provide calories:

- Carbohydrates
- Fats
- Protein

Calories are only part of the food equation. You must also be concerned with what you eat. You may stay lean on 2400 good calories a day and gain weight on 1600 calories of junk food.

The American Heart Association recommends this daily nutrient breakdown, in percent of total calories:

- 50% carbohydrate
- 30% fat
- 20% protein

Individuals who exercise on a consistent basis are recommended this caloric breakdown:

- 55 - 60% carbohydrate
- 15 - 20% fat
- 25% protein

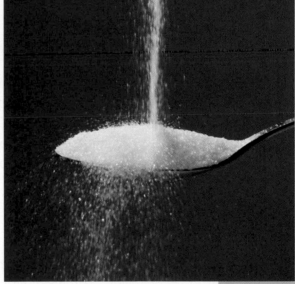

Anyone who exercises frequently needs more carbohydrate storage, because carbs are the body's primary source of energy. The lower fat level decreases your risk of coronary artery disease. The protein level is increased to help build and repair your muscles.

Carbohydrates come in two forms:

1. Simple sugars –

Simple sugars are used for energy almost immediately after consumption. Examples of simple sugars include processed sugar and fruit sugar. Consuming simple sugars alone will not help during endurance exercise.

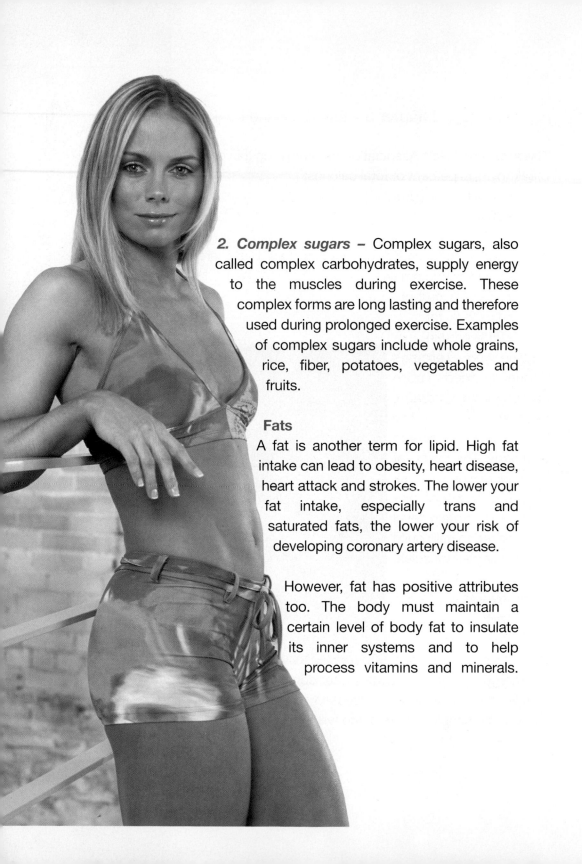

2. *Complex sugars* – Complex sugars, also called complex carbohydrates, supply energy to the muscles during exercise. These complex forms are long lasting and therefore used during prolonged exercise. Examples of complex sugars include whole grains, rice, fiber, potatoes, vegetables and fruits.

Fats

A fat is another term for lipid. High fat intake can lead to obesity, heart disease, heart attack and strokes. The lower your fat intake, especially trans and saturated fats, the lower your risk of developing coronary artery disease.

However, fat has positive attributes too. The body must maintain a certain level of body fat to insulate its inner systems and to help process vitamins and minerals.

Without enough fat, your skin, hair and nails would become brittle and dry. Like carbohydrates, fat also fuels the body during exercise. Your level of fat intake should depend upon your health and fitness goals.

Examples of foods high in fat include cheese, nuts, avocados, cooking oils, butter and cream. It's a good idea to restrict your consumption of these foods. There are three types of fat:

Saturated fat – Saturated fat is the most detrimental to the body because it has the highest number of hydrogen bonds. Overconsumption of saturated fat raises "bad" cholesterol, or LDL, levels and lowers "good" cholesterol, or HDL, causing clogged arteries, heart attacks, strokes and other coronary diseases. You should avoid saturated fat, especially trans fats, aka partially hydrogenated oil.

Polyunsaturated fat – Polyunsaturated fat has fewer hydrogen bonds. Polyunsaturated fat helps raise

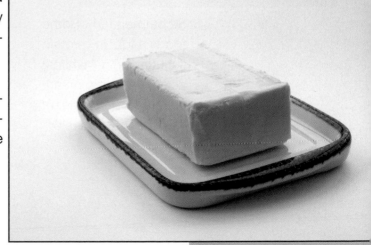

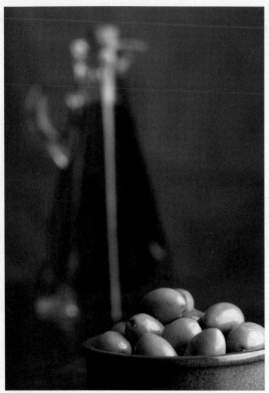

good cholesterol levels and decrease the bad.

Monounsaturated fat – Monoun-saturated fat has even fewer hydrogen bonds than polyunsaturated fat, and is the best of the three. Your fat quota should consist mainly of mono-unsaturated fat, such as olive oil.

Protein

Protein is the building-and-repair material of the human body. Protein is composed of smaller subunits called amino acids, which help to build muscle cells. Your required protein intake depends upon your health and fitness goals. For the average athletic female, a daily intake of .75 grams of protein per pound of body-weight is recommended. Some foods high in protein include egg whites, chicken (white meat), lean beef (red meat), fish, beans and skim milk.

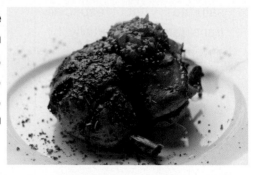

Food Groups

As well as classifying food into nutrient groups, nutritionists have separated them into categories called "food groups." Healthy eating means consuming portions from each group on a daily basis.

Fruits

A great source of vitamins and fiber, fruits are also low in fat. Fresh fruits are much more nutritious than fruits processed with syrups or sugar-sweetened juices. The average adult should eat 2 or 3 servings of fruit each day. The most nutritious fruits are those with deep color, like berries, oranges, and mango.

Vegetables

The average adult should eat 5 to 8 servings of vegetables each day. Vegetables provide vitamins, minerals and fiber and are low in fat. Categories of vegetables include:

- Dark leafy greens like spinach, kale or romaine
- Deep yellow or orange vegetables
- Root vegetables such as yams, beets, and carrots
- Beans
- Squash
- Okra

*Ab*solute Perfection

Grains
This group includes bread, cereal, rice, pasta and corn. These foods are high in carbohydrates. They also contain B vitamins, minerals and fiber. Of all the foods in this group, whole-grain products have the most nutrients. An average adult should eat 6 to 11 servings each day. But stay away from white bread!

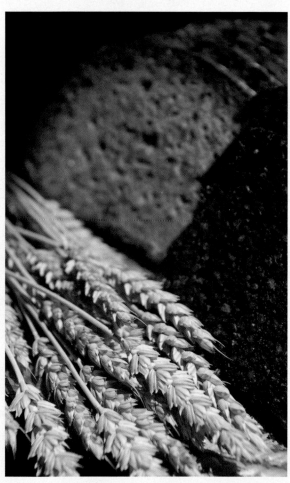

Meats and Meat Substitutes
This food group includes dried beans, nuts and eggs in addition to red and white meat. These groups give you protein, iron, zinc, B vitamins, calcium and vitamin E. Eat 2 or 3 servings from this group per day, or more if you are physically active.

Dairy Products
Yogurt, ice cream and cheese – as well as milk – have lots of calcium. They also contain protein and some vitamins. Most of the items in this group are naturally high in fat. Low-fat varieties have much lower amounts of calories, cholesterol and saturated fat. Eat 2 to 4 servings from this group per day, preferably low-fat varieties.

Fats and Oils

This group contains good fats like olive oil and the omegas, omega 3 in particular, but it also contains bad fats like those found in potato chips, candy bars or pastry. Eat 1 or 2 servings of good fats each day, but limit bad fats to a one-a-week treat. If you are one of the many people who cannot control yourself within the vicinity of these foods, it's best to avoid them entirely.

Try to add good fats to your diet by eating plenty of flax-seed, salmon and grains. Nuts and nut butters are an excellent source, but are quite calorie dense, so limit their quantity.

You should structure your diet to avoid saturated fats.

Chapter 4

Stretch!

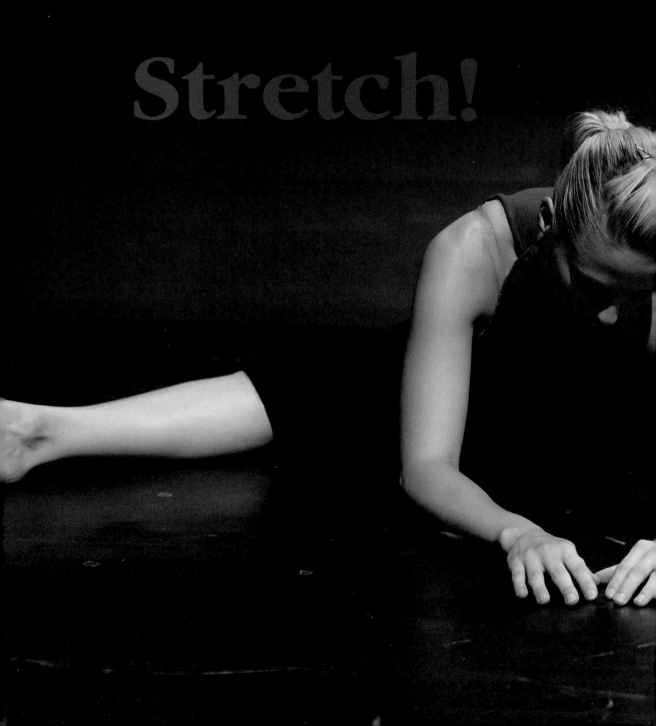

Most readers have seen athletes stretching to prevent injuries and improve their performance. But the act of stretching is beneficial for all of us, not just athletes. We now know that stretching – even on an airplane or at your work desk – promotes circulation, reduces stress, and decreases repetitive-movement injuries. If you have suffered an injury, stretching can rebalance your musculature and help you move with confidence. Improved muscle resilience, coordination and power, and higher energy levels are all benefits of regular stretching. And of course you'll be more flexible!

Flexibility is a key component of a balanced fitness program. Without flexibility training (stretching) you miss out on an important part of overall fitness training. Before exercising, first warm up for five to ten minutes at a low intensity (50 to 60 percent of your maximum heart rate) before stretching. Proceed to doing a cardiovascular activity for at least 20 minutes at an intensity of 50 to 85 percent of your maximum heart rate (see chapter 5 on cardio training). Then cool down for 5 to 10 minutes at a low intensity (50 to 60 percent of your maximum heart rate). Now, because your muscles are very warm, you should stretch all of the major muscle groups.

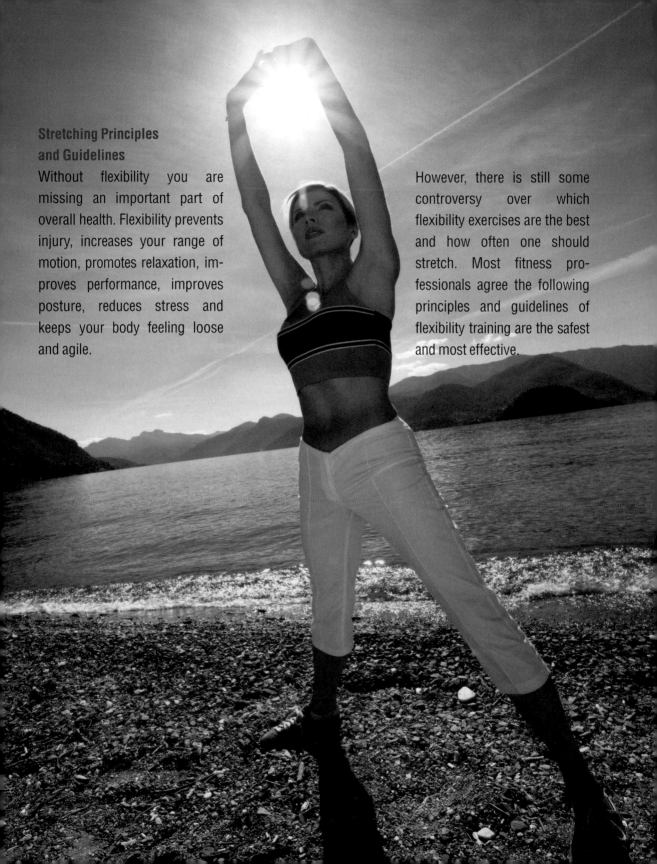

Stretching Principles and Guidelines

Without flexibility you are missing an important part of overall health. Flexibility prevents injury, increases your range of motion, promotes relaxation, improves performance, improves posture, reduces stress and keeps your body feeling loose and agile.

However, there is still some controversy over which flexibility exercises are the best and how often one should stretch. Most fitness professionals agree the following principles and guidelines of flexibility training are the safest and most effective.

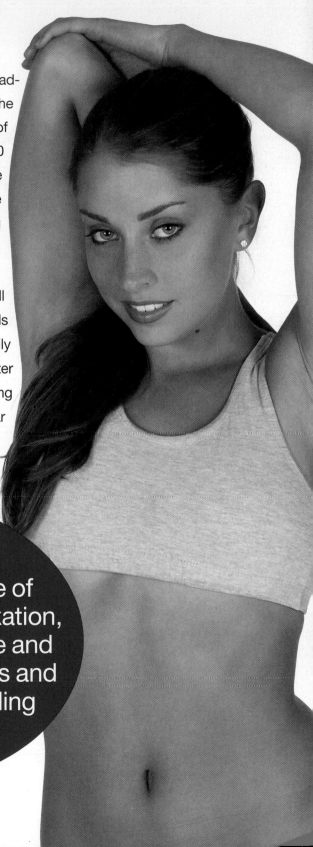

Use Static Stretching

Static stretching involves a slow, gradual and controlled elongation of the muscle through the full range of motion and holding for 15 to 30 seconds in the furthest comfortable position (without pain). This is the first and most important stretching principle.

How often you should stretch is still hotly debated. Most professionals would agree, however, that daily stretching is best during and after exercise sessions. Frequent stretching will help you avoid muscular imbalances, knots, tightness and muscle soreness created by daily activities and exercise.

Flexibility prevents injury, increases your range of motion, promotes relaxation, improves performance and posture, reduces stress and keeps your body feeling loose and agile.

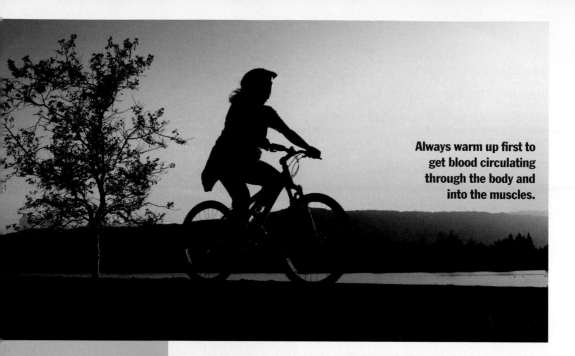

Always warm up first to get blood circulating through the body and into the muscles.

Always Warm Up Before Stretching

Never stretch a cold muscle! A warm muscle is much more easily, and safely, stretched. Always warm up first to get blood circulating through the body and into the muscles. Try stretching an elastic band that has just come out of a freezer. See how quickly it breaks. The same is true for cold muscles. While you probably won't tear a muscle by stretching it, you could suffer a minor muscle strain.

A warmup should be a slow, rhythmic exercise that uses the larger muscle groups. Riding a bicycle or walking works well and provides the body with a period of adjustment between rest and more vigorous activity. The warmup should last about 5 to 10 minutes and should be similar to the activity you are about to do, but at a much lower intensity. Once your muscles are warm, you can then stretch.

42

Stretch Before and After Exercise

We recommend stretching both before and after exercise, each for different reasons. Stretching before an activity (after the warmup) improves dynamic flexibility and reduces the chance of injury. Stretching after exercise ensures muscle relaxation, facilitating normal resting length, circulation to joint and tissue structures and removal of unwanted waste products, thus reducing muscle soreness and stiffness. Body temperature is highest right after cardiovascular exercise or strength training. In order to achieve maximum results, static stretching is highly recommended just after your cardiovascular exercise and during or after your strength training.

Stretch Between Weightlifting Sets

Strength and flexibility training are both important for everyone. Those of you who have trouble finding time to incorporate a strength-training program

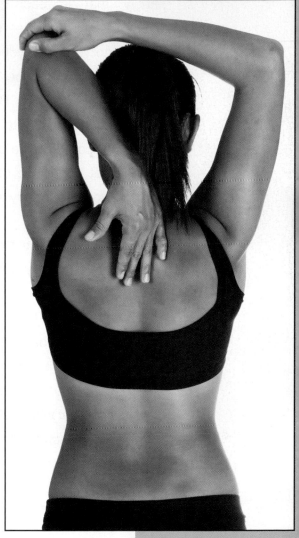

into their lifestyle can combine stretching with strength training. If you have had any experience in strength training, you know that in each exercise for each muscle group you train, you have a certain number of sets, usually 2 to 4. Between each set, you need to rest and let your muscle recover before going on to the next set of repetitions. Well, what better use of your resting time than to stretch the muscle you're currently training?

Never stretch a cold muscle! Always warm up first to get blood circulating throughout the body and into the muscles.

You've just done a set of 10 reps of leg extensions. Now you have to rest, usually about one minute, before doing the next set. This is a great time to stretch your quads. The area is warm and you have time before you start your next set. And stretching requires so little energy that doing it between sets won't interfere with your weight training.

Do your first set with relatively light weight to warm up. Rest for a minute or so, increase the weight and go on to the next set of 10 reps (or whatever your rep goal happens to be). After the second

44

set, your muscles should be warm and ready to be stretched. While resting and before your third set, stretch the muscle you have just trained, remembering the important principles of a static stretch, then proceed to your third and final set. Stretch the muscle one more time. Try stretching a little further. Proceed to the next exercise for the next muscle group. After it is warm, do your stretch for that muscle, and so on. When you have gone through each of your strength-training exercises, you will have stretched each muscle without taking up any more time.

Stretch Before and After Cardiovascular Exercise

Use the static stretching techniques we explained previously. For example, if you walked on the treadmill, you should stretch your quadriceps, hamstrings, calves and

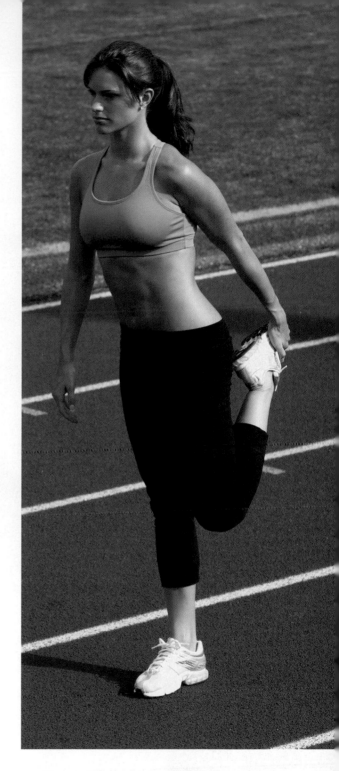

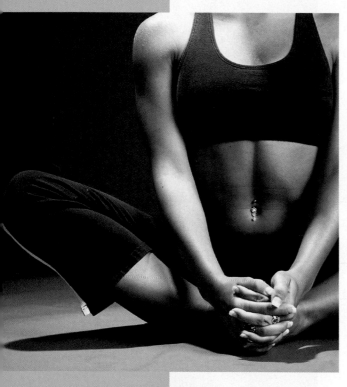

lower back. Proper technique for each stretch is absolutely crucial for achieving maximum effectiveness in any one specific muscle group. In addition to stretching those muscles used in the exercise, now is also a good time to go through a full-body stretching routine, since blood has circulated throughout your entire body and warmed up your muscles.

You now have the knowledge to achieve the results you desire and the benefits your body deserves. Your greatest challenge, however, is not learning new stretching exercises or the proper technique. It's not learning how long to hold the stretch or the best time to stretch. Nor is it deciding when to try new stretching exercises. The greatest challenge facing you at this moment is deciding whether or not you are willing to make the commitment, take action and make flexibility training a priority.

Common Stretches

Hamstring stretch – Stand with feet close together, facing straight ahead. Slowly bend from your hips, your head hanging down. Try to reach the floor but don't go further than you can without feeling pain. You just want to feel a gentle pull in the muscle. Hold the stretch for 20 seconds. Do not bounce!

Achilles' stretch – Stand facing a wall and place one

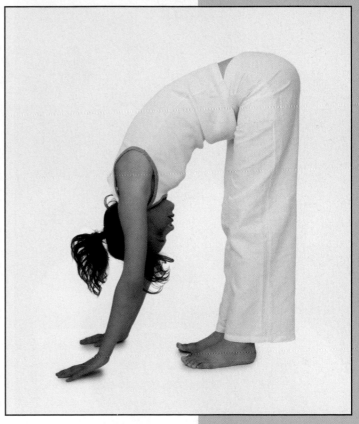

47

Absolute Perfection

leg in front of the other. Bend your front knee and put your hands on the wall. The back leg is straight, with the heel flat on the floor. Lean toward the front knee, keeping the back foot and heel flat. Hold for 15 to 20 seconds. Relax. Repeat with the other leg.

Hip-flexor stretch – Bring one leg forward in a lunge position. Then lower the knee of your rear leg down toward the floor

Groin stretch – Sit on the floor or ground. Put the soles of your feet together, with your knees as close as possible to the ground and pointed outward. Grasp your ankles and hold that position for a count of 10. Relax and repeat three times.

Spread groin stretch – Start in a sitting position with your legs spread apart. Place your hands on the inside of your legs, and try to reach the inside of your ankles. Bend forward from the hips, keeping your knees flat. Hold until you feel tightness on the inside of your legs. Relax, and repeat.

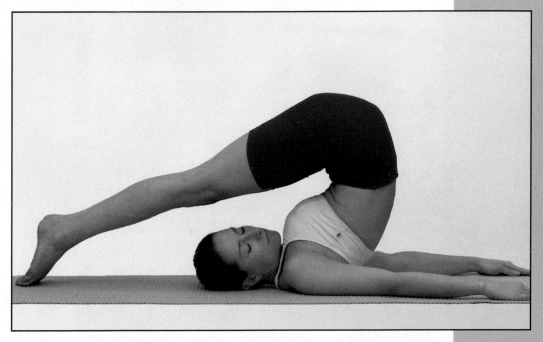

Back stretch – Lie on your back. Raise one leg, grabbing hold of it right by the knee, towards your hamstrings. Slowly pull your knee toward your chest. Keeping your other leg straight and your head on the ground, hold this position for a count of 10. Repeat three times with each leg.

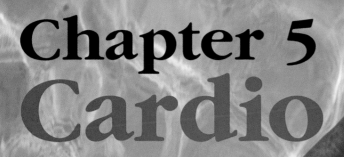

Chapter 5
Cardio

Weight training and stretching are important, but no exercise is as important as cardiovascular training. A weak skeletal muscle will probably only be a nuisance to your daily life but let your heart muscle get slack and see what happens. Of couse, health and fitness go hand in hand with looking great, and nothing burns fat like cardio.

For maximum effectiveness and safety, cardiovascular exercise has specific goals with regard to frequency, duration and intensity. Here are the most important components of cardiovascular exercise. Make sure you understand and implement these components in your training program.

Warming Up and Stretching

One common mistake is stretching before the muscles are fully warmed up. It is important to stretch *after* your muscles are warm (after blood has circulated through them). 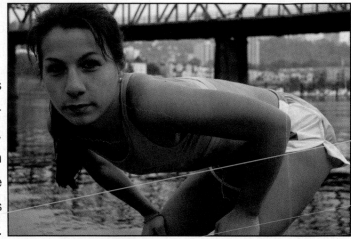 Never stretch a cold muscle. Always **warm up**. A warmup should be done for at least five to ten minutes at low intensity. The warmup is usually accomplished by doing the same activity as the cardiovascular workout but at an intensity of only 50 to 60 percent of maximum heart rate (Figuring out your desired heart rate will be covered later in this chapter.) After five to ten minutes at a relatively low intensity, your muscles should be warm. To prevent injury and to improve your performance, you're best to stretch the primary muscles used in the warmup before proceeding to cardiovascular exercise.

51

Cooling Down

The **cooldown** is similar to the warmup in that it should last five to ten minutes and be done at a low intensity (50 to 60 percent of max HR). After you have completed your cardiovascular exercise and cooled down properly, it is again important to stretch the primary muscles used. Warming up, stretching, and cooling down are important to every exercise session. Not only do they help your performance levels and produce better results, they also drastically decrease your risk of injury.

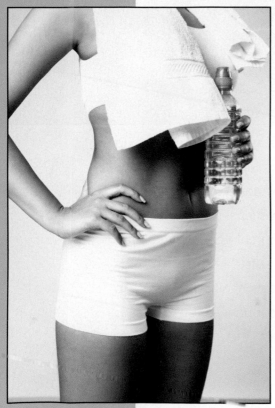

Frequency of Exercise

The first component of cardiovascular exercise is **frequency,** which refers to the number of exercise sessions per week. To both improve cardiovascular fitness and decrease body fat or maintain body fat at optimum levels, you should exercise at least three days a week. The American College of Sports Medicine recommends three to five days a week for most cardiovascular programs. If you are out of shape or overweight and taking part in weight-bearing cardiovascular exercise such as an aerobics class or jogging, you might want to take at least 36 to 48 hours of rest between workouts to prevent an injury and to promote adequate bone- and joint-stress recovery.

Duration of Exercise

The second component of cardiovascular exercise is *duration*, which refers to the time you spend exercising. A cardiovascular session, not including the warmup and cooldown, should vary from 20 to 60 minutes to gain significant cardiorespiratory and fat-burning benefits. Each time you perform cardiovascular exercise try to do at least 20 minutes or more. Why? Because for the first 15 to 20 minutes the body is burning stored sugar (glycogen) as a fuel source. It's the second 15 to 20 minutes that really hits fat deposits.

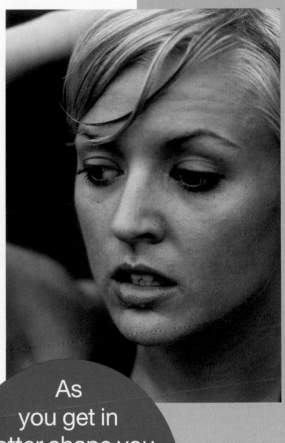

As you get in better shape you can gradually increase the length of your exercise sessions.

53

*Ab*solute Perfection

An obvious reason to exercise longer is to burn more calories. The more calories used up overall, the more stored fat you'll burn. All beginners, especially those who are out of shape, should take a conservative approach and train at relatively low intensities (50 to 70 percent max HR) for 10 to 25 minutes. As you get in better shape, you can gradually increase the length of your exercise sessions.

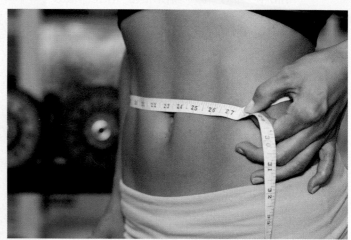

An important precaution is to gradually increase the duration before you increase the intensity. When beginning a walking program, for example, be more concerned with increasing the number of minutes of the exercise session before you increase the intensity by speeding up or by walking uphill. It's the old "first we crawl, then we walk, then we run" adage.

After you finish your warm-up and your cardiovascular exercise, you should stretch the main muscles used. For example, after cycling, stretch your quadriceps, hamstrings, calves, hips and lower back. After using the rowing machine, stretch your legs, back, biceps and shoulders.

Determining the best intensity level for cardiovascular exercise

Over the years exercise physiologists have tried to come up with ways to measure workout intensity. Some involve "numbers and percentages" while others are no more complicated than having a "chat." Although the mathematicians among you may gravitate toward numbers, the "talk test" does have its place.

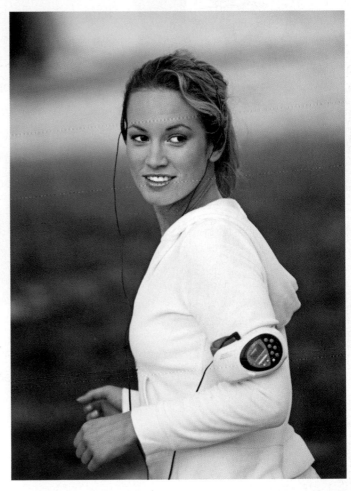

Your Heart Rate by the Numbers

There are two ways to check your heart rate during exercise. The most accurate is to purchase a heart-rate monitor. It will give you feedback on a digital watch, telling you exactly what your heart rate is at a specific time in the exercise session. Many home and commercial cardio machines have built-in heart monitors. Some are straps that plug into the machine, while others are built into the machine's handles.

The other way to determine your heart rate is by palpating (feeling) the carotid artery, the temporal artery, or the radial artery. The easiest site to locate the heart rate is either the carotid or the radial artery. The carotid artery may be felt by gently placing your index finger on your neck, between your collarbone and jaw line. Palpating the radial artery is done by placing your index and middle fingers on the inside of your wrist just under the thumb.

When you're taking your heart rate you measure it in beats per minute (counting the number of beats for 60 seconds). For convenience, many people take their pulse for 10 seconds and multiply that number by six. If in 10 seconds you counted 20 beats, that would mean your heart rate was 120 beats per minute (bpm). Keep in mind that the longer the time interval used, the more accurate the results will be. For example, counting your heart rate for 30 seconds and then multiplying that number by two will give a slightly more accurate reading than counting for 10 seconds and multiplying by six.

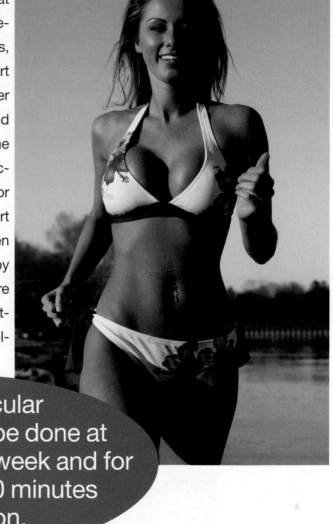

Cardiovascular exercise should be done at least three times a week and for a minimum of 20 minutes per session.

*Ab*solute Perfection

Heart Zone Training

How do you know if you are training too intensely or not intensely enough for what you want to achieve? One method is to use what's called the **target heart rate zone**. Refer to the chart below. The top of the chart reads "Maximum Heart Rate," which is 100 percent of your heart rate (the fastest your heart will beat). This number is different for everyone. To use heart-zone training you must first determine your maximum heart rate (max HR).

You can determine your max HR in either of two ways. One way is to use the age-predicted max HR formula, whereby you subtract your age from 220. So, if you are 40 years old, your predicted max HR would be 180 bpm. The other method, which is much more accurate and more individualized, is actually having

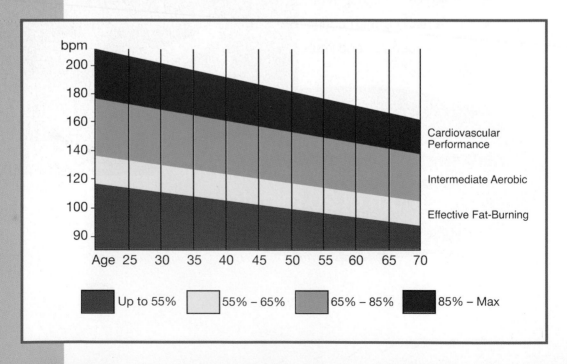

a medical or fitness professional administer a max HR test for you. The test is usually conducted on a stationary bicycle or treadmill for several minutes and requires very hard work. Thus, only those cleared by a physician should take this test, and only trained professionals should administer it.

Once you have determined your max HR, you will need to decide at which zone you wish to train. As you can see, there are different training zones separated by increments, each having different characteristics and benefits.

Healthy Heart Zone

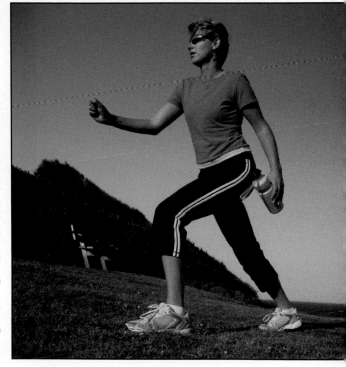

The first zone is the Healthy Heart Zone (in purple). This means the heart will achieve rates up to 55 percent of max HR. This is the easiest and most comfortable zone in which to train and is best for people who are just starting an exercise program or have low functional capacity. Those of you who are walkers likely train in this zone.

59

Although this zone has been criticized for not burning enough total calories and for not being intense enough to get great cardiorespiratory benefits, it has been shown to help decrease bodyfat, blood pressure and cholesterol. Training in the Healthy Heart Zone also decreases the risk of degenerative diseases and presents a low risk of injury, especially for those new to exercise. In this zone energy burned is made up of five percent protein, 10 percent carbohydrates and a whopping 85 percent fat.

Fat-Burning Zone

The next zone is the Fat-Burning Zone (yellow), which is 55 to 65 percent of your max HR. Once again, 85 percent of calories burned in this zone are fats, 5 percent are proteins and 10 percent are carbohydrates. Studies have shown that in this zone you can condition fat mobilization (getting fat out of your cells) while conditioning fat transportation (getting fat to muscles). Thus, you are training your fat cells to increase the rate of fat release and training your muscles to burn fat. In this zone you get the same benefits as in the Healthy Heart Zone when training at 55 percent, but you are now slightly increasing the total number of calories burned and providing more cardio respiratory benefits. You burn more total calories at this zone simply because it is more intense.

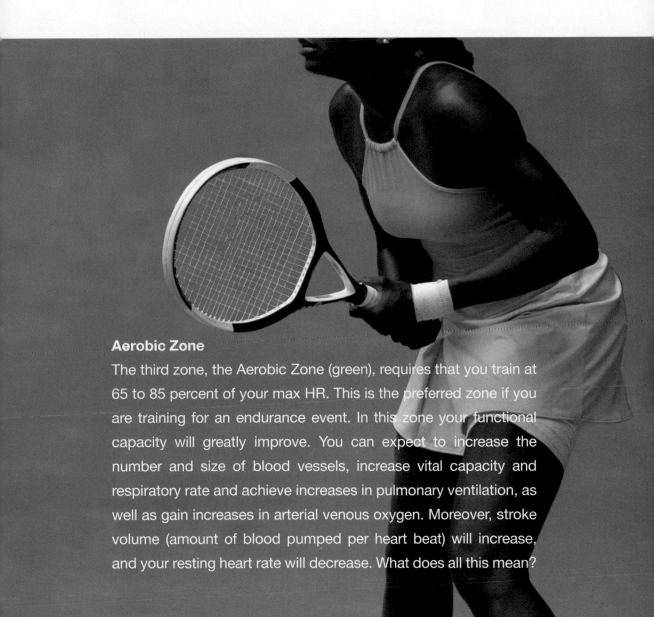

Aerobic Zone

The third zone, the Aerobic Zone (green), requires that you train at 65 to 85 percent of your max HR. This is the preferred zone if you are training for an endurance event. In this zone your functional capacity will greatly improve. You can expect to increase the number and size of blood vessels, increase vital capacity and respiratory rate and achieve increases in pulmonary ventilation, as well as gain increases in arterial venous oxygen. Moreover, stroke volume (amount of blood pumped per heart beat) will increase, and your resting heart rate will decrease. What does all this mean?

*Ab*solute Perfection

It means your cardiovascular and respiratory system will improve and you will increase the size and strength of your heart. In this zone 50 percent of calories burned are from 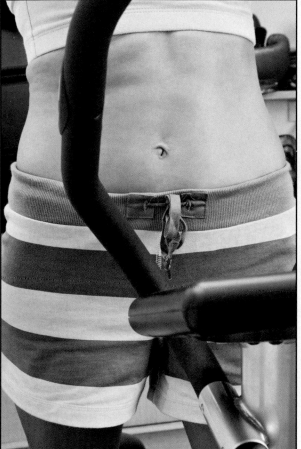 carbohydrates, 50 percent are from fat, and less than one percent is from protein. And, because intensity is increased, there is also an increase in the total number of calories burned.

Cardiovascular Performance Zone

The next training zone is called the Cardiovascular Performance Zone, which is anything above 85 percent of your max HR. Benefits include an improved VO2 maximum (the highest amount of oxygen one can consume during exercise) and thus an improved cardiorespiratory system, as well as a higher lactate tolerance ability – which means your endurance will improve and you'll be able to fight fatigue better. Since the intensity is extremely high, more calories will be burned than within the other three zones. Although more

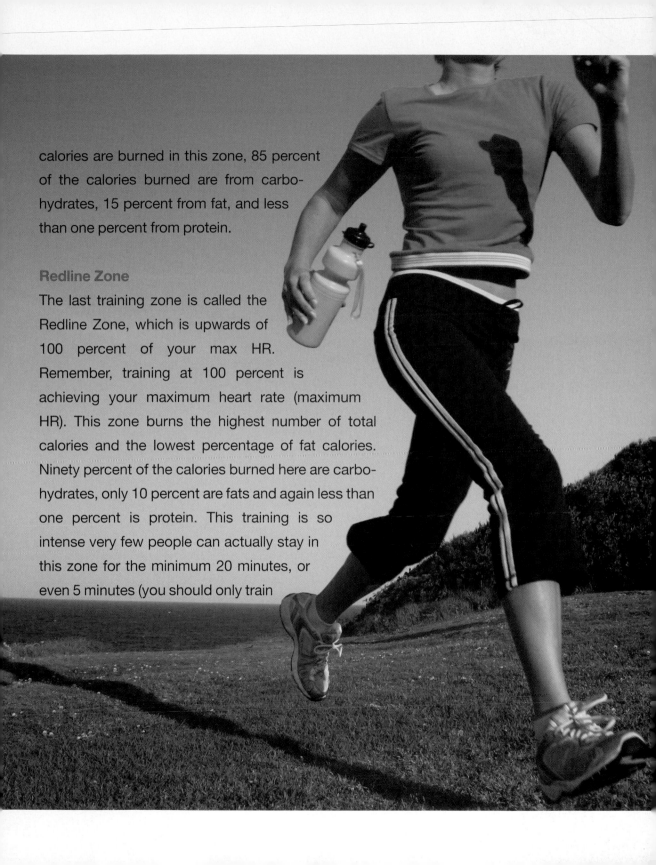

calories are burned in this zone, 85 percent of the calories burned are from carbohydrates, 15 percent from fat, and less than one percent from protein.

Redline Zone

The last training zone is called the Redline Zone, which is upwards of 100 percent of your max HR. Remember, training at 100 percent is achieving your maximum heart rate (maximum HR). This zone burns the highest number of total calories and the lowest percentage of fat calories. Ninety percent of the calories burned here are carbohydrates, only 10 percent are fats and again less than one percent is protein. This training is so intense very few people can actually stay in this zone for the minimum 20 minutes, or even 5 minutes (you should only train

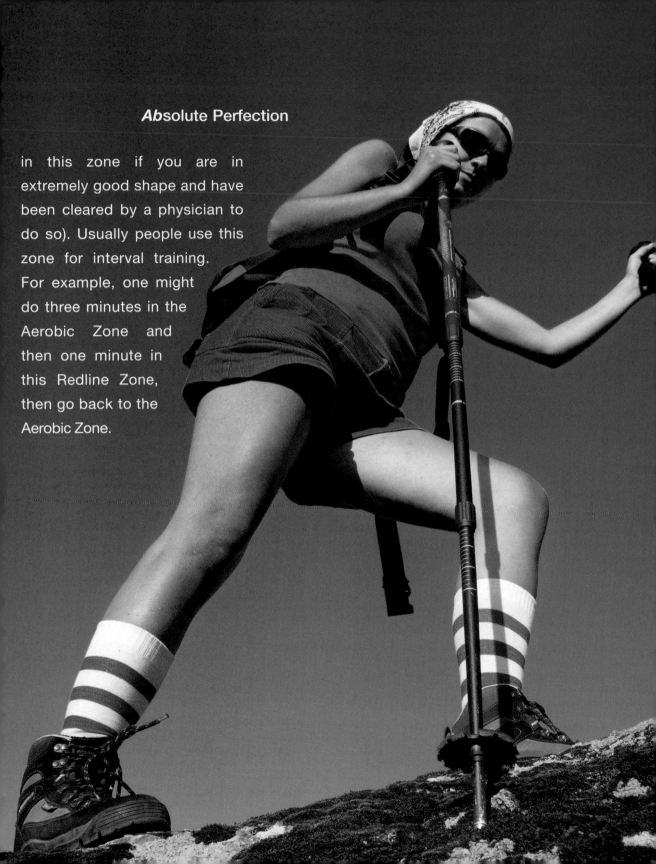

Absolute Perfection

in this zone if you are in extremely good shape and have been cleared by a physician to do so). Usually people use this zone for interval training. For example, one might do three minutes in the Aerobic Zone and then one minute in this Redline Zone, then go back to the Aerobic Zone.

Your Innermost Feelings

Although the Target Heart Rate Zone method is probably the most common, a simpler system for measuring intensity exists. It's called the Borg Rating of Perceived Exertion (RPE) and it's another way of determining how hard you are working.

Perceived exertion is how hard you *feel* your body is working. It is based on the bodily sensations a person experiences during physical activity, including increased heart rate, increased respiration, or breathing rate, increased sweating and muscle fatigue. Although this is a subjective measure, a person's exertion rating may provide a fairly good estimate of the actual heart rate during physical activity.

Practitioners generally agree a perceived exertion rating of between 12 and 14 on the Borg scale suggests physical activity is being performed at a moderate level of intensity. During physical activity, use the Borg Scale to assign numbers to how you feel. Self-monitoring how hard your body is working can help you adjust the intensity of the activity by speeding up or slowing down your movements.

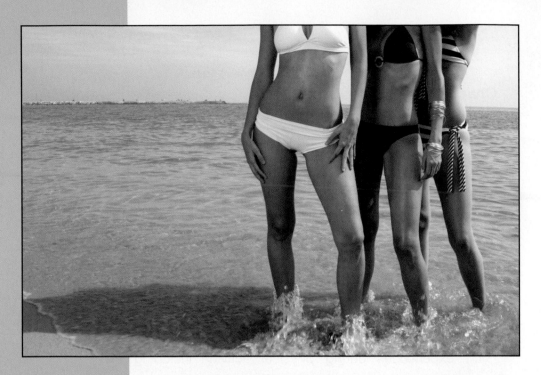

Through the experience of monitoring how your body feels, it will become easier to know when to adjust your intensity. For example, a walker who wants to engage in moderate-intensity activity would aim for a Borg scale level of "somewhat hard" (12 to 14). If she describes her muscle fatigue and breathing as "very light" (9 on the Borg scale) she would want to increase her intensity. On the other hand, if she felt her exertion was "extremely hard" (19 on the Borg scale) she would need to slow down her movements to achieve the moderate intensity range.

Research has determined that a high correlation exists between a person's perceived exertion rating multiplied by a factor of 10 and the actual heart rate during physical activity. So a person's exertion rating may provide a fairly good estimate of the actual heart rate during activity. For example, if a person's rating of perceived exertion (RPE) is 12, and 12 x 10 = 120; so the heart rate would be approximately 120 beats per minute. Of course, this calculation is only an approximation of heart rate. The actual heart rate can vary quite a bit depending on age and physical condition. The Borg Rating of Perceived Exertion is the preferred method to assess intensity among those individuals who take medications affecting heart rate or pulse.

The next time you exercise try rating your level of exertion. This rating should reflect how heavy and strenuous the exercise feels to you, combining all sensations and feelings of physical stress, effort and fatigue. Do not concern yourself with any one factor, such as leg pain or shortness of breath but try to focus on your total feeling of exertion. Look at the rating scale on the next page. It ranges from 6 to 20, where 6 means "no exertion at all" and 20 means "maximal exertion." Choose the number that best describes your level of exertion while you are engaging in an activity. You can use this information to speed up or slow down your movements to reach your target range.

Paying close attention to how you feel while you exercise will help you stay within your target heart rate range.

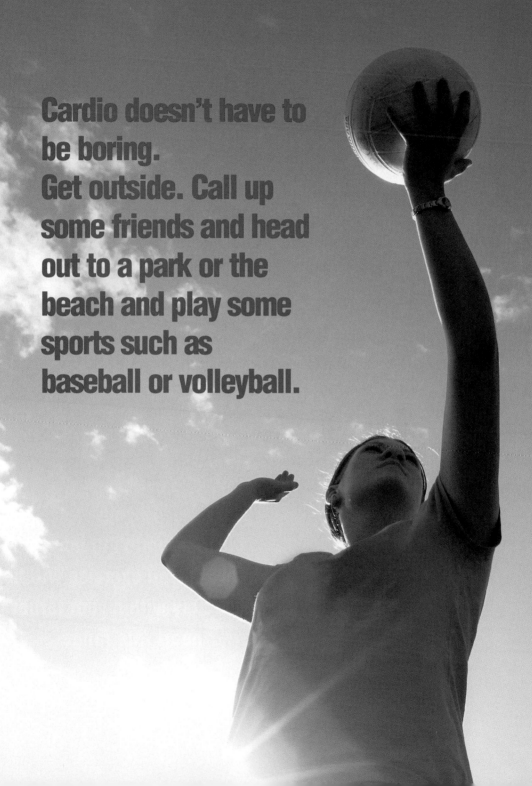

Cardio doesn't have to be boring.
Get outside. Call up some friends and head out to a park or the beach and play some sports such as baseball or volleyball.

Level of Exertion

6	No exertion at all
7	
7.5	Extremely light
8	
9	Very light
10	
11	Light
12	
13	Somewhat hard
14	
15	Hard (heavy)
16	
17	Very hard
18	
19	Extremely hard
20	Maximal exertion

Try to appraise your feeling of exertion as honestly as possible, without thinking about what the actual physical load is. Your own feeling of effort and exertion is important, not how it compares to the level of others. Look at the scales and descriptions and then rate your activity level.

69

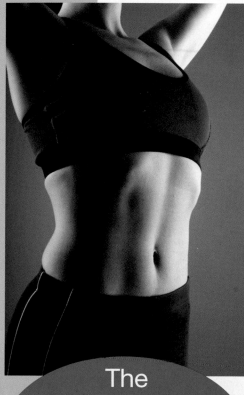

The next time you exercise try rating your level of exertion.

Notes:

• A rating of 9 denotes "very light" exercise. For a healthy person, that would be like walking slowly at your own pace for a matter of minutes.

• 13 on the scale is "somewhat hard" exercise but it still feels good to continue.

• 17 is a "very hard," very strenuous level of exertion. A healthy person can still go on but he or she really has to push it. Exercise feels very heavy and is tiring.

• 19 on the scale is an extremely strenuous exercise level. For many people, this is the most strenuous exercise they have ever experienced. For most this level is too intense for continued exercising. Even if they could somehow get to this intensity level, remaining there would be too dangerous.

Talking About Your Heart Rate

For those who hated high-school math and don't want to bring numbers into an exercise activity, a far simpler rating system is available. It's called the "talk test" and it's as simple as it gets. A person who is active at a light intensity level should be able to sing while doing the activity. One who is active at a moderate intensity level should be able to carry on a conversation comfortably while engaging in the activity. If a person becomes winded or too out of breath to carry on a conversation, the activity can be considered vigorous. If she is gasping for air and unable to talk, then she is most likely working at an extremely high intensity level beyond the high end of the aerobic zone and into the anaerobic zone. This level is fine for short periods of time but unless you are at an elite level of fitness or a top sports competitor, you probably want to ease off.

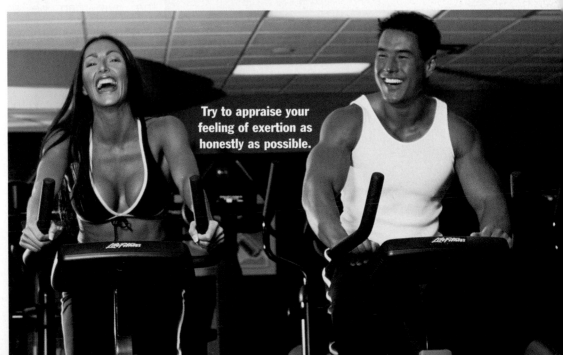

Try to appraise your feeling of exertion as honestly as possible.

Cardio Exercises – *Burn, baby burn!*

Cardio exercise doesn't have to be a boring, tedious, time-consuming experience. With the right approach, cardio can be an *enjoyable* activity to help reduce bodyfat and improve cardiovascular fitness. Let's look at a few simple tips to help make your cardio workout more fun. Remember to consult your doctor before starting any diet and exercise plan.

One of the best ways to make your routine more fun is to mix up your choice of cardio activities. Cardio doesn't have to be restricted to indoors, either. Take advantage of the good

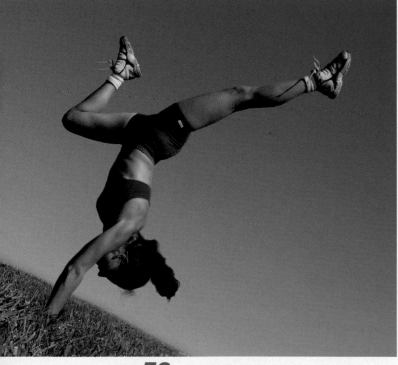

weather. Go outside and do some running, in-line skating, or cycling. Getting out of the gym can be a refreshing change. Explore your neighborhood or some other part of town with which you're less familiar. One fun cardio adventure is to take public transit to a certain point and then work

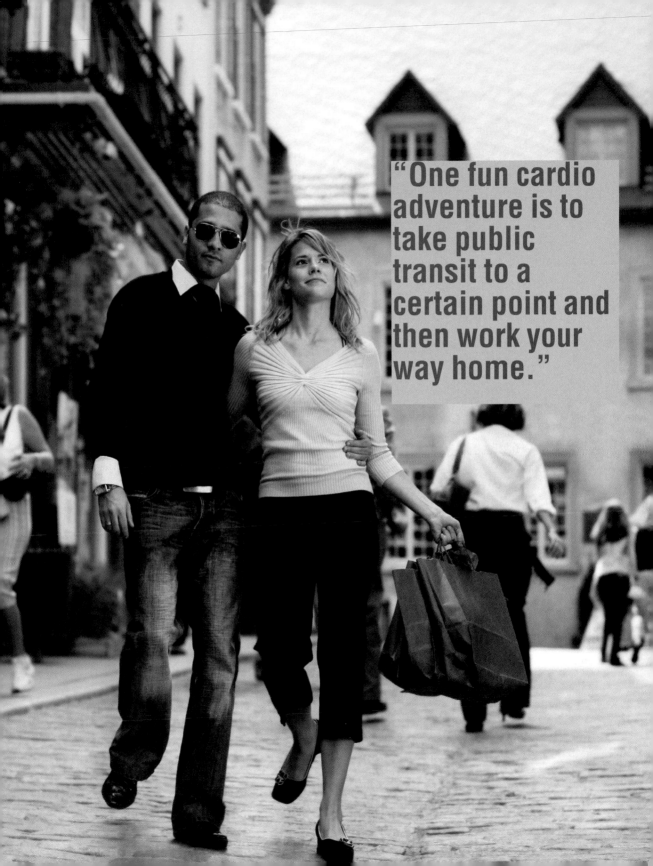

"One fun cardio adventure is to take public transit to a certain point and then work your way home."

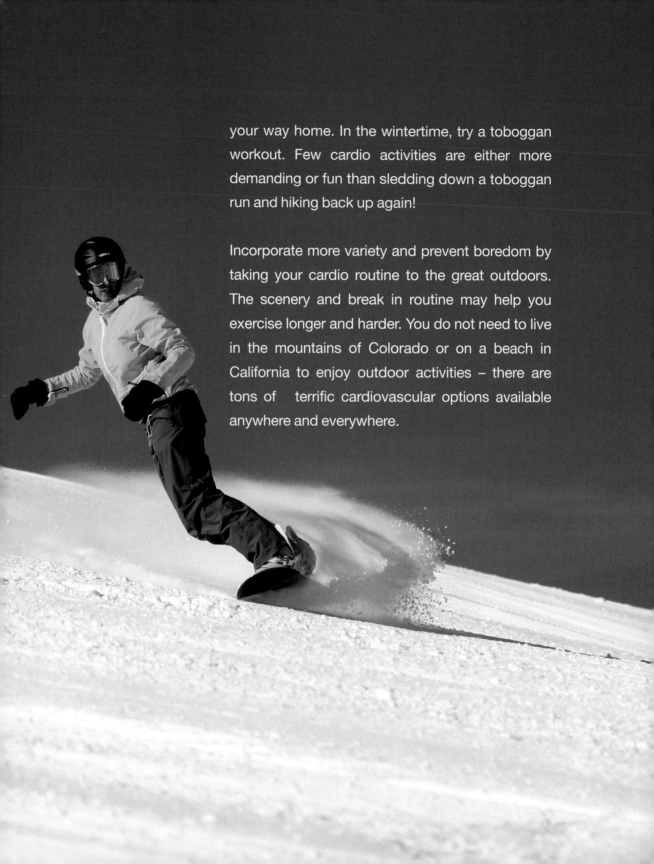

your way home. In the wintertime, try a toboggan workout. Few cardio activities are either more demanding or fun than sledding down a toboggan run and hiking back up again!

Incorporate more variety and prevent boredom by taking your cardio routine to the great outdoors. The scenery and break in routine may help you exercise longer and harder. You do not need to live in the mountains of Colorado or on a beach in California to enjoy outdoor activities – there are tons of   terrific cardiovascular options available anywhere and everywhere.

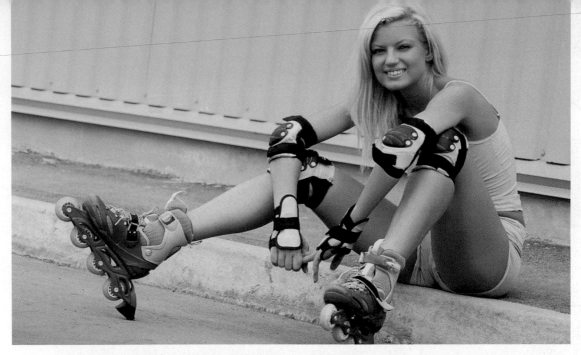

Another excellent cardio exercise is running. Bike paths make a great place to run – they are safe from traffic, often lined with water fountains, and if they are hilly, can help build power and speed. To spice up your outdoor runs, find a moderately steep hill with consistent footing. Run up the hill at a steady pace and then jog down. Rest and repeat. Another twist on your outdoor running routine is to do tempo runs. Here you alternate minutes of running at a steady pace with seconds of sprinting. Hiking is another option for an enjoyable outdoor workout.

With the right approach cardio can be an enjoyable activity, both to help reduce body fat and to improve cardiovascular fitness.

Swimming develops endurance and upper-body strength. The pool at your health club is ideal if you are

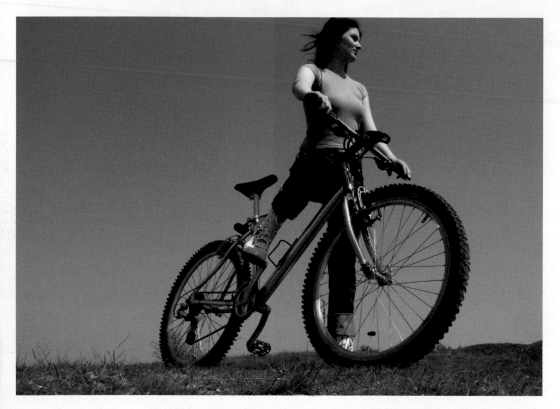

swimming year-round but can become boring lap after lap. Find a local lake that permits swimming and has lifeguards on duty and take the plunge! Lakes are good for swimming longer distances since you do not constantly have to stop and turn. For safety, never swim alone or without a lifeguard present.

Are you an avid user of the stationary bike at the gym? Pull your bicycle out of the garage and find a local trail to ride. Dedicated bike trails are great because they are closed to cars and you can cycle for long distances in a safe, scenic environment. For an even greater endurance test, ride your bike to a forest preserve trail that is slightly hilly. The hills will challenge you and provide an effective interval workout. You can also do "out-and-backs" – bike for a certain distance, note your time and try to improve that time on the way back. No matter what type of bike workout you choose, be sure to wear a helmet and follow the path rules. In winter months, instead of being bothered by the snow and ice, take advantage. Those paths that you cycle and run on are great for cross-country skiing.

Also consider participating in sports for recreation. Grab a friend and hit the tennis court or head to the beach to play volleyball. With both activities, make an effort to run down every ball to strengthen leg muscles and build endurance.

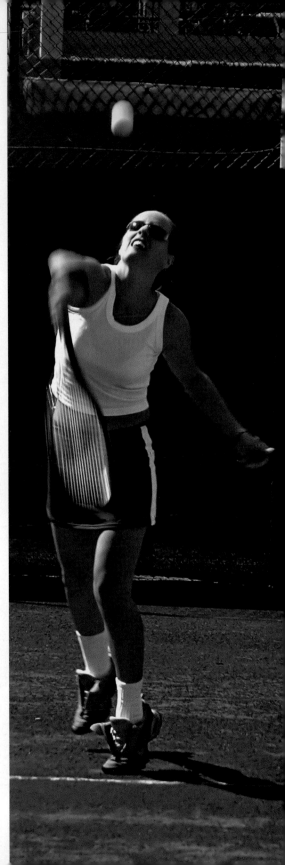

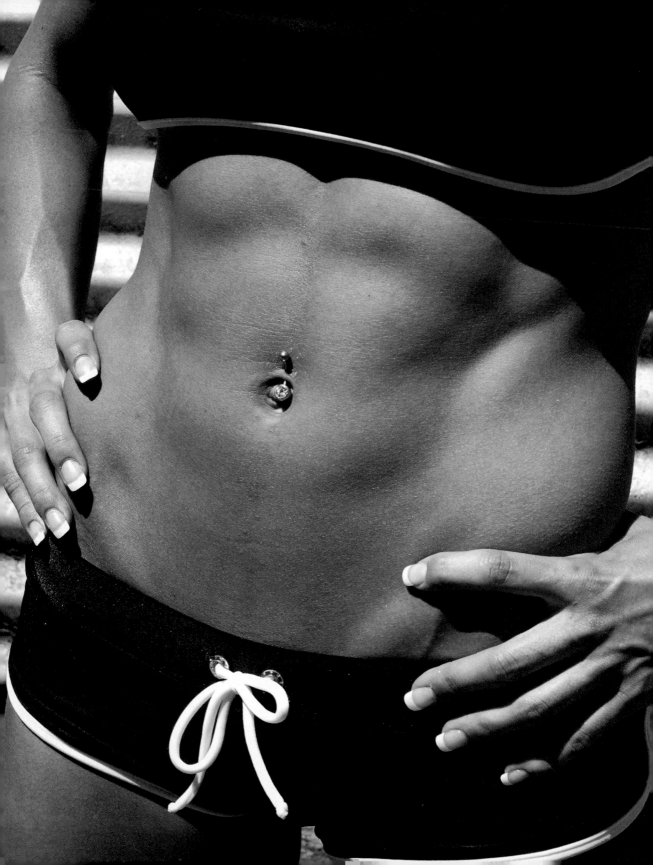

Chapter 6

Down
to the
Crunch

O ne of the many myths of weight loss is that abdominal exercises promote fat loss. This could not be further from the truth, as can be attested by millions of Americans who have purchased and used abdominal exercise machines in an effort to lose weight. The only way to attain fat loss is through improved eating habits and regular exercise. Abdominal exercise machines do nothing more than strengthen and tighten abdominal muscles. If, and it's a big if, some people who buy those TV gizmos do in fact lose weight, it's usually because they follow the diet and exercise program accompanying the product. Performing hundreds of "ab rolls" does virtually nothing to get rid of the spare tire around your midsection. Many people begin exercising with an expectation of losing weight quickly, not realizing their efforts are being

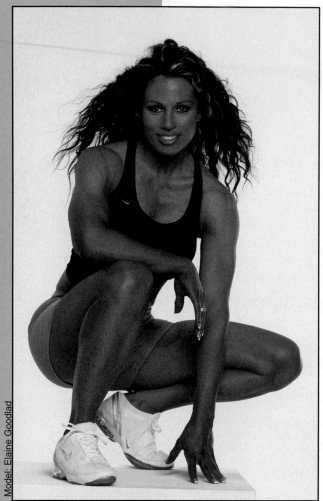

Model: Elaine Goodlad

wasted. Where do these misconceptions come from?

The answer is simple. People in general don't understand the facts about fat loss and exercise … and manufacturers of abdominal exercise machines know this. They are only too happy to step forward and take advantage of the average person's desperation to lose weight. It is against the law for companies to outright lie about performing abdominal exercises to attain fat loss, so in fine print you will always see that a healthy nutritional plan should be used in conjunction with the product for best results. If you do indeed lose weight by using their abdominal exercise machines it will be as a result of the diet and not the exercise. Put another way, the consumer has just spent $50-$100 for a diet and exercise plan. There are far cheaper ways to get the same results.

Abdominal muscles – up, down, all around

Before you can properly train the abdominals you need to know a little about their anatomy. What we call the abdominals is actually a group of several muscles: the rectus abdominis, transverse abdominis and the external and internal obliques. The serratus, though technically not part of the abdominals, adds a finished look to the area when developed. The abdominal muscles sit on the front and sides of the lower half of the torso, originating along the rib cage and attaching along the pelvis.

Functions

Rectus abdominis – These muscles flex the spine (bringing the rib cage closer to the pelvis). This flexing is seen in the abdominal crunching movement.

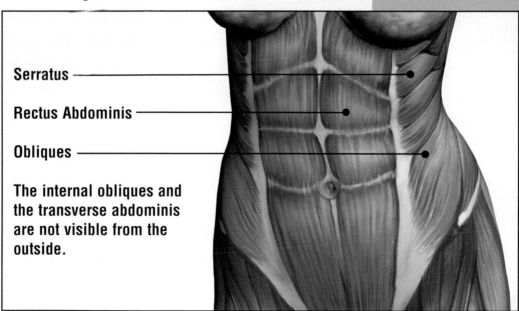

Serratus

Rectus Abdominis

Obliques

The internal obliques and the transverse abdominis are not visible from the outside.

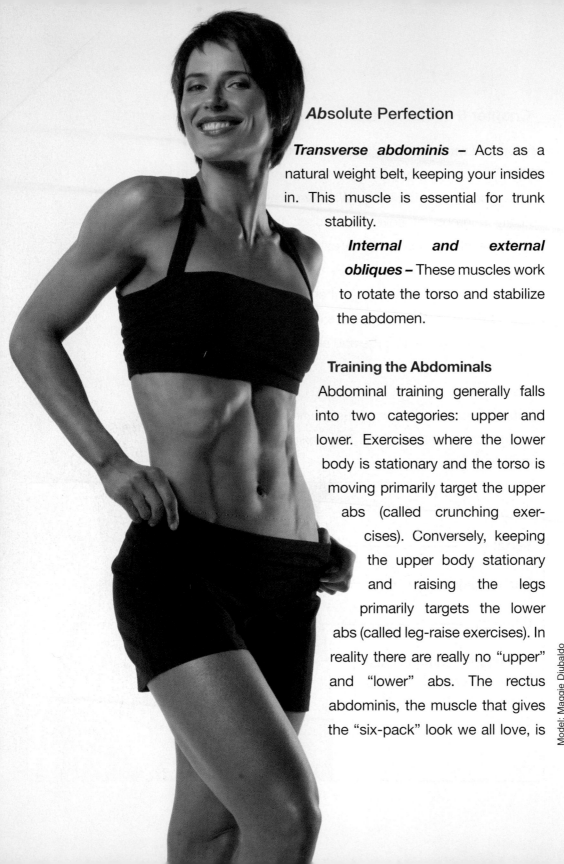

Absolute Perfection

Transverse abdominis – Acts as a natural weight belt, keeping your insides in. This muscle is essential for trunk stability.

Internal and external obliques – These muscles work to rotate the torso and stabilize the abdomen.

Training the Abdominals

Abdominal training generally falls into two categories: upper and lower. Exercises where the lower body is stationary and the torso is moving primarily target the upper abs (called crunching exercises). Conversely, keeping the upper body stationary and raising the legs primarily targets the lower abs (called leg-raise exercises). In reality there are really no "upper" and "lower" abs. The rectus abdominis, the muscle that gives the "six-pack" look we all love, is actually one muscle. It just looks like six muscles because of the tendons that run down the middle and to the sides, dividing it into six little bricks and a long lower part.

Many kinesiologists say you can't separate the upper and lower abs. However, you can shift the emphasis. You can't totally isolate one region of the abs but you can target it. This is why you should include both crunching and leg-raise movements in your abdominal workouts.

Upper Abdominals

The upper abdominal region tends to develop easily because the muscle in the area is dense and responds well to intense exercise. Another reason the upper abdominals seem to develop more easily than the lower abdominals is that less fat accumulates there.

The upper abdominals receive the most stimulation during movements that flex the spine from the upper torso (i.e. crunches). When performing these exercises, focus on pulling your chest down

> The only way to lose body fat tissue located directly on top of the abdominal muscles is to follow a fat-burning diet capable of accomplishing such a task.

*Ab*solute Perfection

toward your hips. To reduce the stress on the lower back and reduce the amount of hip flexor involvement, try to keep your knees slightly bent and your lower back pressed to the floor. Keep your chin tucked in and your hands across your body. Be sure not to pull the upper body forward by pressing on the back of your head with your hands. This position not only reduces the stress on your abdominals but can also easily cause damage to the upper spine.

Lower Abdominals

As you'll quickly discover, development of the lower abdominal region is a much greater challenge. Fat tends to accumulate in the lower abdominal region faster than in the upper, especially in women. You may be lean all over your body but hold five to ten extra pounds in the lower abdominals. Does that mean you

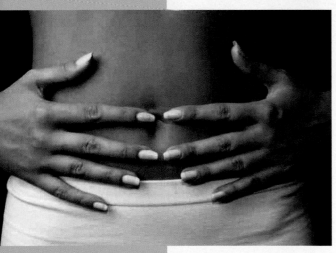

should give up on building the lower abdominals? Of course not. It just means you have to be a little bit more creative and persistent when it comes to training the "lowers."

The best way to train the lower abdominals is with exercises that bring your pelvic area toward

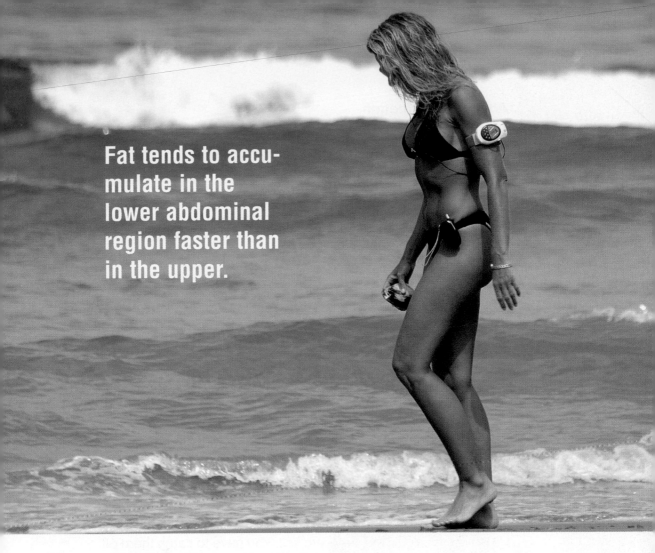

Fat tends to accumulate in the lower abdominal region faster than in the upper.

your chest. The most productive movements are the reverse crunch and the leg raise, and the hanging leg raise is probably best of all. Don't simply raise your legs off the floor. Try to consciously curl your pelvis toward your chest. Because of the limited range of pelvic motion, the hip flexors will want to take over and dominate most lower-ab exercises. You must pay close attention to strict form and always squeeze as much as you can out of each repetition.

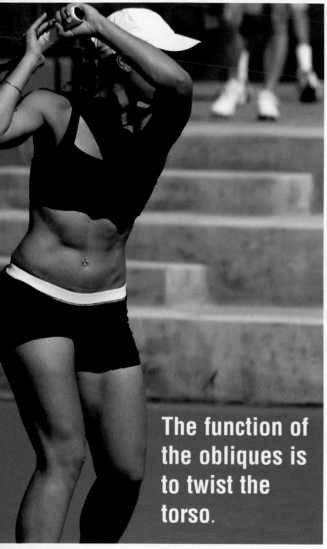

The function of the obliques is to twist the torso.

The Obliques

The obliques rest on either side of your abdomen. Their function is to twist your torso. While you do want to keep them toned, you do not want to spend too much effort on the obliques, as building them up will only give your waist a thick appearance.

Abdominal Training – General Principles

The abdominal muscles are masters of adaptation. Your gains will quickly plateau after only a few sessions using the same exercises. You have to catch them off guard, so to speak. The best way to accomplish this is to rotate the exercises regularly. What's more, even slight variations in a movement can help recruit different muscle fibers. The end result is better abdominal development. The variety will also keep your workouts more interesting.

86

How Often?

The debate rages about how often to train the abdominals. For some people nothing less than every day is acceptable. Others suggest the abdominals should be treated like any other muscle group – two or three sessions per week, maximum. We lean more toward the latter. Muscle tissue is actually broken down during exercise, not built up. The resting period is when growth and development takes place. If you interfere with the recovery process you could impede your progress.

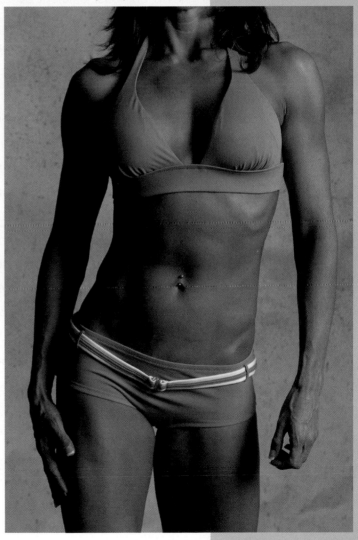

87

Abdominal Exercises
Situps

We are going to start this section by discussing perhaps the most well-known but *least* efficient ab exercise there is ... but hold on, we have an important reason for doing so. Situps have been around for ages and just about everybody has tried them at some point. No doubt many readers have fond memories of junior-high gym class where your partner held your feet to the floor and you had to raise up and touch your knees. *Oh, the pain. Oh, the anguish! Oh, the* foolishness *of it all.*

That's right, situps, despite their advanced age, are virtually useless for targeting the abdominal muscles. Why? Because most of the movement is being carried out by the hip flexors. The abdominals only move, or bend the torso, 10 to 12 inches in the average person. Once your shoulders are that far off the floor, the hip flexors take over and raise your torso the rest of the way. More importantly, just picture the stress being placed on your vertebrae. The human spine was not meant to be squished up this way.

Situps work mainly the hip flexors and not the abs.

So what does all this mean? It means we are not going to recommend doing situps – ever! There are many far safer and more effective abdominal exercises you can perform. Please read on.

1. Crunches

Crunches are perhaps the direct opposite of situps in that they are the safest and most effective abdominal movement available. They have become the most commonly performed abdominal exercise. This is a super isolation exercise for the entire rectus abdominis area as well as the intercostals. Best of all, you can perform crunches just about anywhere.

How to do them:

1. Lie flat on your back. If you like, you can place your calves on a

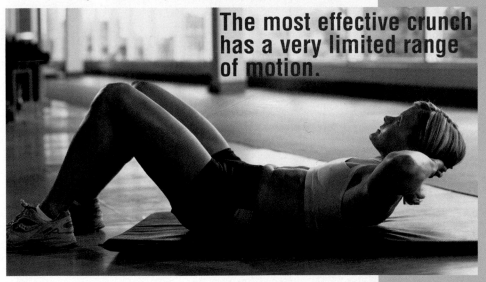

The most effective crunch has a very limited range of motion.

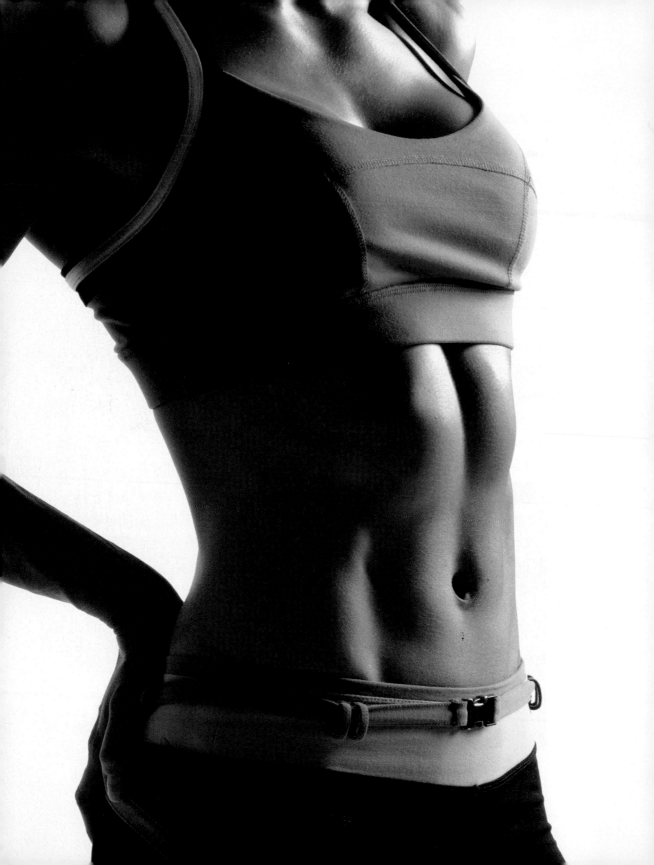

flat bench, chair, or table. Your hamstrings should be at lease 90 degrees to the floor.

2. Place your hands behind your head with fingers interlaced.

3. Perform the following movements simultaneously:

> a. Pull your hips from the floor using your lower abdominal muscles.
>
> b. Raise your shoulders and upper back using your upper abdominal muscles.
>
> c. Force your shoulders in, moving them toward your hips.
>
> d. Exhale.

4. Hold the contracted position for a slow count of 1 to 3 seconds.

5. Keep repeating this movement until fatigued.

2. Lying Leg Raises

Lying leg raises work the whole abdominal region, but since the lower body is doing the moving, the lower abs receive the most stimulation.

How to do them:

Lie on your back with your hands palms down under your buttocks. Raise your legs about 12 inches off the floor and hold them there. Now, conciously trying to use only your lower

> The best way to train the lower abdominals is to use exercises that bring your pelvis toward your chest.

abdominals, raise your legs another 15 to 20 inches. Do this by tilting the pelvis instead of lifting the legs with the psoas (hip flexors). Make sure your knees are slightly bent.

3. Hanging Leg Raises

This relatively new abdominal exercise is rapidly gaining popularity in gyms. Hanging leg raises place intense stress on the entire rectus abdominis, especially the lower part. The intercostals are also tested during this movement.

How to do them:

1. Hang on a chinning bar using an overhand grip with arms straight at shoulder width apart.

2. Bend your legs about 15 degrees. Keep them bent and relaxed during the entire exercise.

3. Raise your feet upward in an arc until they are a bit higher than level with your hips. Make sure to use your abdominal muscles to perform this action.

4. Hold this contracted position for a slow count of one or two seconds.

5. Return slowly to starting position.

6. Repeat repetitions until fatigued.

7. To increase the intensity you can raise your feet higher during each repetition or perform this exercise with ankle weights.

4. Reverse Crunches

Reverse crunches are a superb exercise for working the lower abs.

How to do them:

1. Lie flat on your back with legs extended. Draw your legs in to form an L-shape with your torso. You can bend your knees a bit.

2. Lower your legs almost to the floor – in fact, you can touch the floor with your toes – and raise again.

3. Keep going until failure.

5. Roman-Chair Situps

This is a newer version of the situp. The Roman chair apparatus has been used extensively in gyms for about 30 years. This exercise involves the entire rectus abdominis, although more stress is placed on the upper half.

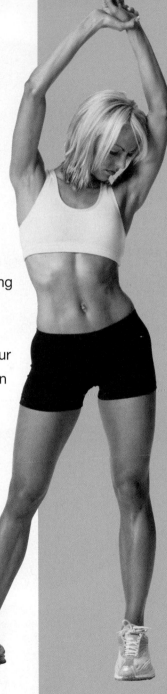

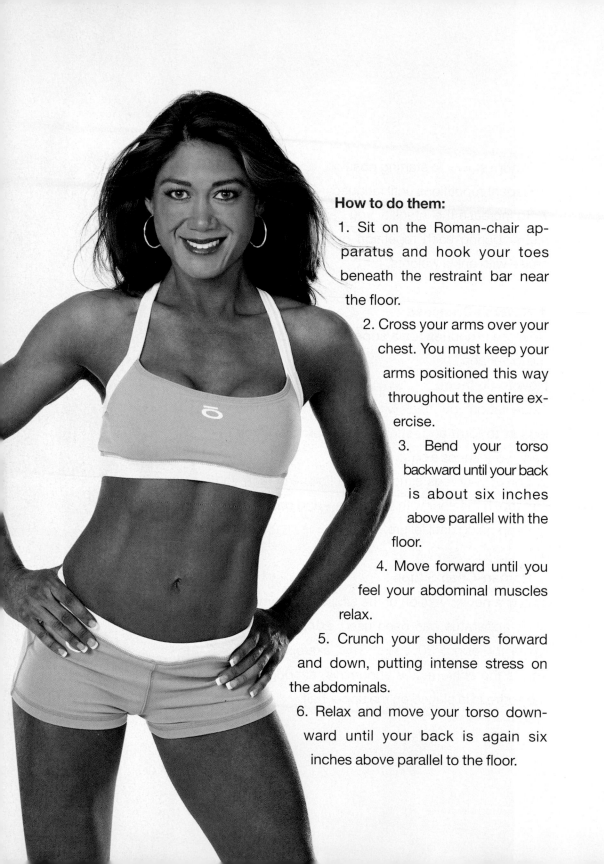

How to do them:

1. Sit on the Roman-chair apparatus and hook your toes beneath the restraint bar near the floor.

2. Cross your arms over your chest. You must keep your arms positioned this way throughout the entire exercise.

3. Bend your torso backward until your back is about six inches above parallel with the floor.

4. Move forward until you feel your abdominal muscles relax.

5. Crunch your shoulders forward and down, putting intense stress on the abdominals.

6. Relax and move your torso downward until your back is again six inches above parallel to the floor.

7. Continue until you have completed the desired number of repetitions.

8. You can add resistance by propping the front end of the Roman chair up on a large block of wood, or by holding a weighted barbell plate behind your head. For a real challenge, you may want to do both.

6. Bench Knee-Ins

This exercise hits the entire abdominal area and is very good for core strength. It targets the lower abs slightly. Those with weak backs may want to avoid this exercise. That being said, it does help strengthen the lower back area, so you can put it to good use.

How to do them:

Sit across a bench, as shown. Reach around and hold the bench behind you for stability. Stretch your legs out until your feet are not quite touching the floor and your knees are not quite straight. Lean back. Draw your knees up toward your torso while you sit up.

95

7. Incline-Board Leg Raises

Leg raises are a common abdominal exercise, nearly as old as situps but far more effective. This movement places primary stress on the lower half of the rectus abdominis, although the muscle fibers of the upper rectus abdominis are recruited as well. Secondary stress is also placed on the intercostal muscles.

How to do them:

1. Lie on your back on an inclined ab board or bench, with your head toward the raised end.

2. Grasp the end of the upper bench with your hands to stabilize your body.

3. Bend your legs 15 to 20 degrees or until you feel your back relax.

4. Use your abdominal muscles to raise your feet in an arc to a position directly above your head.

5. Lower your feet in a return arc until they clear the bench.

6. Repeat until you have completed the desired number of repetitions.

7. Add resistance by raising the incline angle of the bench or by holding a light dumbell between your feet.

Swiss Balls

Physiotherapists have been using stability balls for years for core-region development, and crunches on a Swiss ball have been proven to stimulate the abdominal region more than any other exercise.

These balls force the body to adapt to unusual positions. Unlike floor exercises, Swiss ball movements involve the recruitment of many stabilizing muscles, which aid in the development of strength, flexibility and alignment of the core region.

You can get a better range of motion on a Swiss ball than on the floor by lowering your torso about 30 degrees below parallel before starting the movement. Set your buttocks on the ball and roll backward until you feel a deep stretch all the way down to your lower abs. As you curl up, roll forward again until the ball is once more just under your shoulder blades. Essentially, each rep includes a back-and-forth roll to enhance the range of motion.

97

Chapter 7

Weight Training
Build Muscle, Lose Fat!

Firing Up Your Furnace

You can think of your metabolism as the furnace for your body. When your furnace, or metabolism, is running efficiently, it will burn calories and fat to give your body the energy it needs to function. As we get older, our metabolism requires less fuel to work efficiently – due in part to a reduction in muscle mass. The only way to prevent a sluggish metabolism is to preserve and build muscle tissue … and the only way to do that is through strength training.

The more muscle mass your body has, the more fat it will burn, the more calories you can consume in a day without weight gain and the less baggage you'll hold around your waist. Working out with weights or performing weight-bearing exercises helps the

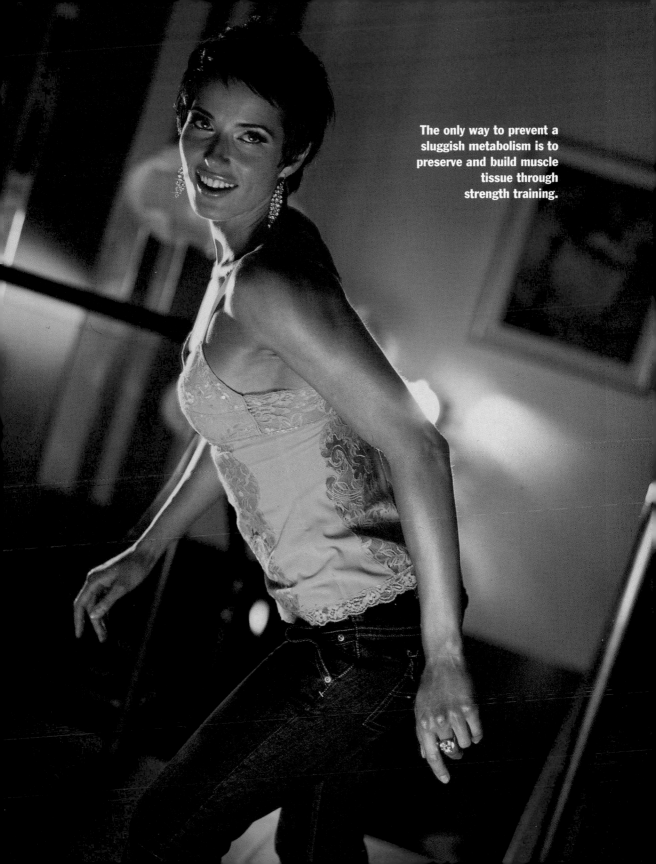

The only way to prevent a sluggish metabolism is to preserve and build muscle tissue through strength training.

*Ab*solute Perfection

body to build muscle tissue. Regular aerobic activity, including walking, jogging and biking, also builds muscle, but only a small amount. Aerobic activity is especially good at burning fat, however, so significant and consistent fat burning – likely the type of weight loss you're hoping to achieve – will occur if your fitness routine includes both building lean muscle tissue and regular aerobic activity.

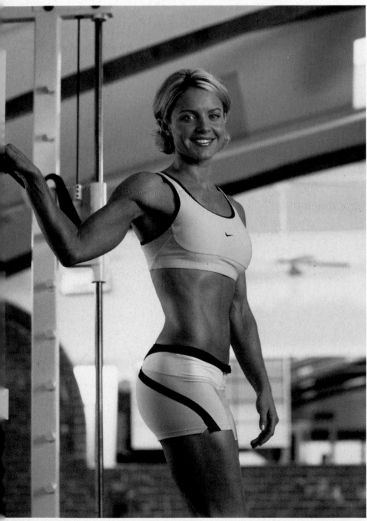

No Bodybuilder's Body

Many women have a fear of weight training because of a mistaken notion that they will end up looking like Arnold Schwarzenegger in his earlier days. The reality is, women simply do not naturally bulk up like that. If you've seen photographs of female bodybuilders who look like muscular men with makeup on, you should keep in mind that they not only have to work extremely hard to look that way, they also had to take steroids. Women simply do not bulk up just from weight training. However, the models you see in the photos throughout this book all weight train. I'd be willing to bet you wouldn't mind looking like them!

While muscle is far denser than fat, and therefore takes up much less room per pound, it also uses up far more calories than fat does. One pound of muscle uses approximately 50 calories a day to maintain, whereas a pound of fat uses only about two calories a day. So an extra 10 pounds of muscle, which will simply make you look more toned, will also burn an additional 500 calories every single day. An extra 10 pounds of fat will do nothing but make you look chubby.

Many women don't feel comfortable working out in a gym, especially if they are significantly overweight. The good news is, you can get a great workout right in your very own home.

Training at Home

Some women, especially those who are considerably overweight, do not feel comfortable working out in a gym. Others may not want to spend the money. While you may eventually want to join a gym,

*Ab*solute Perfection

you don't have to. In fact there are numerous advantages to working out at home. For starters, you can work out whenever it's convenient for you. You set "the gym hours," so to speak. If that's before work in the morning, great. Or perhaps you'd like to train during the evening news. Training at home offers the ultimate in flexibility.

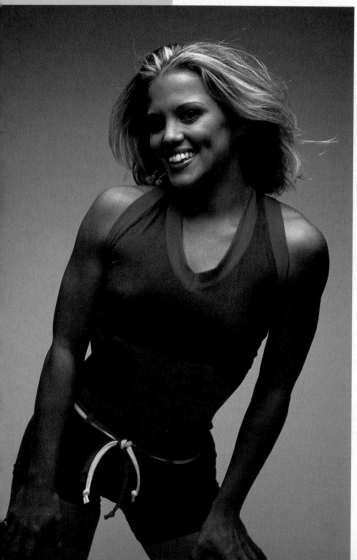

Another advantage of working out at home is that there is no waiting for equipment. Many gyms are crowded, especially from 5 pm to 8 pm. In a crowded gym you may take twice as long to complete your workout as you do at home.

Do you have a favorite type of music? Most people do. Gyms usually pipe in radio music, which is fine if it's a station you enjoy. But if not you'll have to endure it for your entire workout. At home you are the music master and

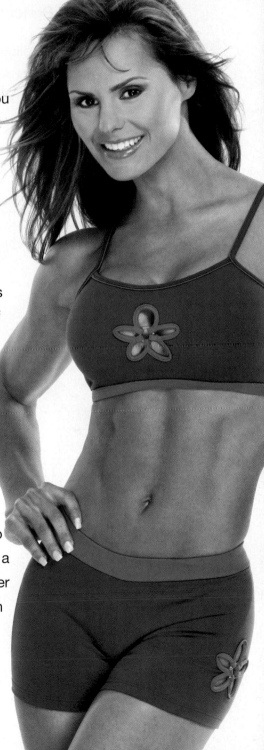

can listen to whatever you please. And you can wear whatever you like to exercise at home. You can even work out in the nude if you choose to!

A final benefit of hitting the weights at home is that you can go right from your last set to the shower. You don't have to worry about such things as bringing a change of clothes and shampoo, or picking up a case of athlete's foot.

With the exception of a few dumbbell exercises, all of the following movements can be performed without any equipment. As for dumbbells, if you don't have a set you can pick them up for mere pennies at a flea market or used-sports-equipment store. You might want to invest a few additional dollars and purchase a skipping rope, which can be bought for under $20, and a barbell set and adjustable bench for about $150.

Model: Timea Majorova

*Ab*solute Perfection

Perform the following metabolism-boosting strength-training program three or four times per week. To keep your heart rate elevated, rest only about 30 seconds between sets. That way you are not only building muscle but also getting a mini-cardio workout in the process. The end result is increased calories burned both during and after your workout. Take a good look at your belly bulge, because it's about to disappear!

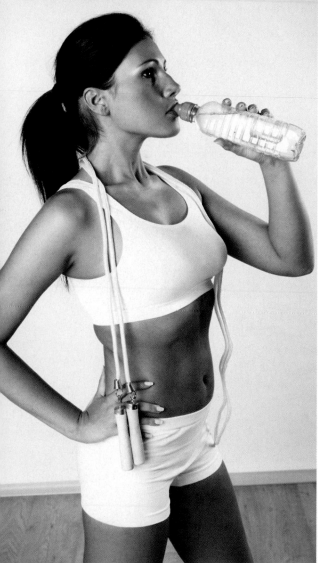

Introductory Weightlifting Terms

Like most forms of physical activity, weightlifting has its own vocabulary. Don't worry, it's nothing fancy, and rest assured there will be no exam at the end of this chapter!

Reps – If the cell is the basic unit of life, the rep is the basic unit of weightlifting. *Rep* is short for *repetition,* and simply means the execution of one complete movement of an exercise. If you were to get down on the floor and perform 10 pushups, that would be considered 10 reps. Deep, or what?

Sets – You can say you did a group of 10 reps, but weight trainers use another term for group and that's "set." A set is a group of reps. The most common, and arguably the most productive number of reps in a set is 8 to 12.

For maximum size and strength some people lift extremely heavy weights for 4 to 6 reps. For general light toning and conditioning, 15 to 20 reps would be better. For most people, however, 8 to 12 reps per set seems to work best, developing both strength and muscle, which helps you burn calories.

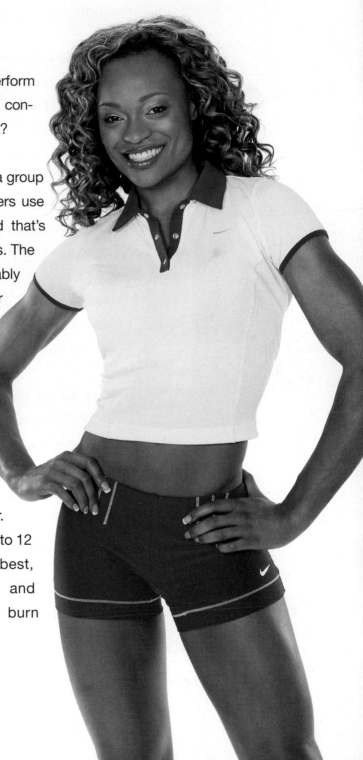

Model: Alicia Marie

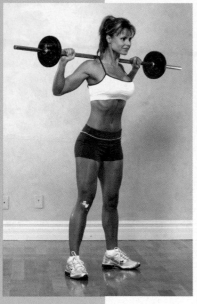

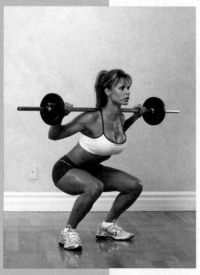

Tempo – Tempo is nothing more than a fancy word for rep speed, and describes the length of time it takes for the up, down and pause during a set. Of an infinite number of tempos, the most common is as follows: Raise the weight slowly, over two seconds, and then lower it in about one second. Others do the opposite, raising the weight quickly and lowering it slowly. As both raising and lowering contribute to effectiveness, we suggest doing a slow-up and slow-down sequence. Try a two-seconds-up, two-seconds-down tempo.

For many exercises it makes sense to pause at the top and bottom of the exercise. A one-second pause will go a long way toward keeping your technique honest, as it's easy to speed things up and use momentum to cheat. If you were to express this in numerical terms it would be "2-1-2-1."

2-1-2-1 – The first two means you raise the weight in two seconds. Then you pause for one second (the first one), lower in two seconds (the second two) and pause for another second (the second one). Don't get too hung up on the numbers. It's pretty easy to estimate one and two seconds. When you are performing your exercises, just make sure you are going at a steady pace and not racing to complete the set.

Training to failure – Training to failure means choosing a weight that allows you to perform a given number of reps and no more. For example, if you were training 12 reps in a set, you would pick a weight that just barely allows you to get 12 reps – you would be physically incapable of performing that 13th rep. In other words you "failed" at the 12th rep.

Muscle is far denser than fat, so you may weigh the same amount but be two sizes smaller. Don't just go by the scale. Make sure you get out the tape measure to find out how you are really progressing.

Time between sets – How long to rest between sets is an individual preference. As with the number of reps per set there is an "average" time – 60 seconds. If you are trying to get an extra bit of cardio stimulation from your workout, as you probably are if you want to lost fat, you might want to reduce the time to 20 or 30 seconds. Conversely, powerlifters may wait two to three minutes between sets.

Since 60 seconds allows enough time to catch your breath without cooling down, it's a good time interval to use.

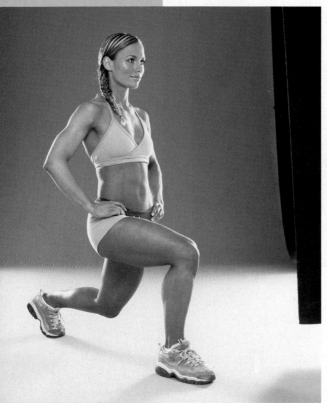

Exercise Descriptions
Thighs
Lunges
How to Perform
Rest a barbell on your shoulders or hold dumbbells in your hands. Slowly step forward and downwards with one leg until there is a 90-degree angle at the knee. Your trailing leg should always have a slight bend at the knee. Return to the standing, upright position.

What they work: Lunges work the thighs and glutes, but the hamstrings come into play.

Modifications: You can do a "walking lunge," in which you keep going from one leg to the other, but instead of stepping back you continually step forward. You need a large area to do this in. Many people perform the walking lunge outside.

Hamstrings
Stiff-Leg Deadlifts

How to perform: Hold a barbell in both hands or a dumbbell or water container in each hand and, with the knees bent slightly, bend forward until the dumbbells (or containers) are just short of touching the floor. Rise back up until the torso is fully erect. Even though the name says "stiff-leg" you should never lock the legs completely. Doing so would place excess pressure on the lower-back ligaments. Also, don't bounce at the bottom of the exercise. Again, you'd be increasing the risk of injury to the lower back.

What they work: Stiff-leg deadlifts are an excellent way to hit the hamstrings. They also work the spinal erectors (lower-back muscles) and glutes.

Modifications: If you have good flexibility try performing the exercise while standing on a platform, such as the bottom step on a flight of stairs.

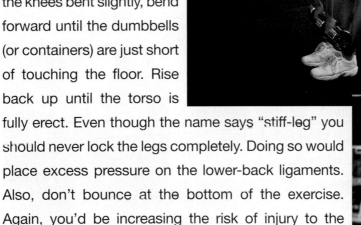

109

*Ab*solute Perfection

Calves
One-Leg Calf Raises

How to perform: Hold a dumbbell or similar weight in one hand and stand on the bottom step of a staircase. Hold the rail with your free hand and rise up as far as you can on your toes using the foot on the same side of the body as the weight you are holding. Stretch down as far as comfortably possible. Repeat for the other leg.

What they work: One-leg calf raises, as the name suggests, work the calves – both the lower soleus and upper gastrocnemius.

Modifications: If you don't have access to stairs, you can stand on a thick piece of wood. Even a beefy textbook will work.

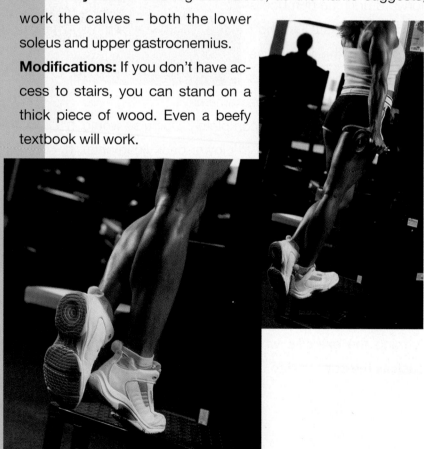

Chest

Dumbbell Presses

How to perform: Grab a pair of dumbbells and lie back on a flat bench. Position the dumbbells so they are facing forward, i.e. they form a straight line. With your forearm kept straight, lower the dumbbells until your upper arm is just slightly below parallel with the floor. Return to the starting position by pressing the dumbbells upward and inward to just short of touching. Always keep the weights under control, particularly as you lower them. Drop too fast or bounce at the bottom and you place considerable stress on the shoulder joints.

What they work: Dumbbell presses are one of the best exercises for targeting the chest muscles. They also bring the front shoulders and triceps into play.

Modifications: If you don't have access to a flat bench you can perform dumbbell presses lying on the floor. Of course your range of motion will be limited – you won't be able to lower your arms below parallel. If you have access to an adjustable bench, you can perform incline dumbbell presses. The exercise is done the same way but the increased angle of the bench shifts more of the stress to the upper chest.

One pound of muscle burns 50 calories a day. One pound of fat burns only two calories a day. Build muscle to burn fat.

111

*Ab*solute Perfection

Pushups

How they are performed:
Kneel down on the floor and position your hands shoulder width apart with the fingers pointing forward. Extend your legs until your weight is resting on your toes. Using your arms and chest, push your torso away from the floor until your arms are just short of locked out. Lower yourself by bending at the

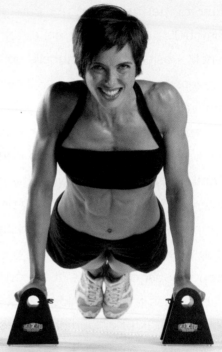

elbows until your nose is an inch or two from the floor. Keep your legs straight at all times.

What they work: Pushups have been performed for thousands of years and remain one of the most effective non-

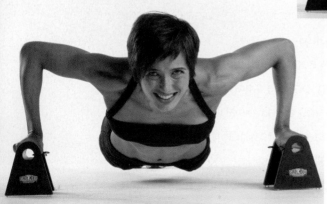

equipment methods of targeting the chest muscles. They also bring the front shoulders and triceps into play.

Modifications: If you don't have the strength to do full pushups, try doing them from your knees (i.e. instead of balancing your weight on your toes you balance on your knees). Conversely, when standard pushups become too easy, try elevating your feet. You can use the first or second step of a stairway, or if you're really ambitious, try placing your feet on a chair. Not only will this position make the exercise more difficult, it also shifts much of the stress to the upper chest, as in incline pressing exercises.

Back

Chinups

How they are performed: With a slightly wider than shoulder-width grip, grab an overhead chinning bar or lead pipe. You can also purchase a bar that fits in a doorway. With your torso leaning back slightly, pull yourself up until your chin is in line with the bar. Lower down to just short of having your arms locked out straight.

What they work: Chinning is another age-old exercise yet to be surpassed by any modern piece of gym equipment. Chinups stimulate just about the whole back region (lats, teres, rhomboids, rear shoulders, spinal erectors), as well as the biceps and forearms.

Modifications: Many people find chins to be quite difficult. Try the assisted chinning machine at a gym, or use a chair to take some of your weight.

113

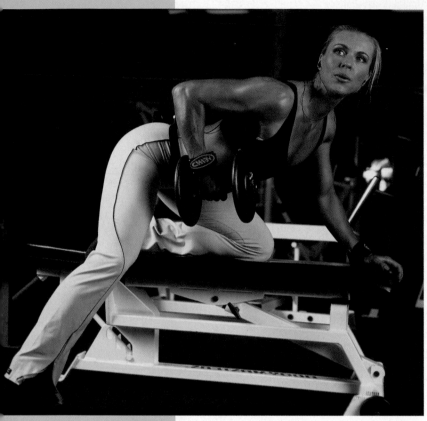

One-Arm Rows
How to perform:

Grab a dumbbell and lean forward, placing one hand on a bench or chair. Pull the dumbbell upward until your upper arm is parallel with the floor. Lower the dumbbell to just short of lockout. With dumbbell rows the key is to keep your body still. Move only your arm. You should not have to twist the spine or bounce up and down with the torso. Concentrate on using your arms just as if they were hooks – try to feel your back muscles do the work.

What they work: One-arm rows work just about the entire back region while the forearms and biceps also play a major role.

Modifications: For extra back support you can place one knee on the bench or chair as well. If you are stuck for time, try lying face down on the bench and performing the exercise with both arms at once.

114

Shoulders
Lateral Raises
How to perform:

With your legs shoulder width apart and knees slightly bent, raise a pair of dumbbells outward and upward until your arms are parallel with the floor. Return to the starting position so the dumbbells are together in front of your body. Always keep a slight bend at the elbows while doing this exercise to help reduce stress on the shoulder joint. Also, don't rock your torso back and forth to lift the weight. If you need to do this to lift the dumbbells, you are using too much weight. You'll likely use only three to five pounds to begin, and probably never more than ten.

What they work: Done properly, lateral raises almost totally isolate the side shoulders. The front and rear shoulders and trapezius play a secondary role.

Modifications: For total control and isolation, try performing the exercise one side at a time by grabbing a wall corner or chair for support.

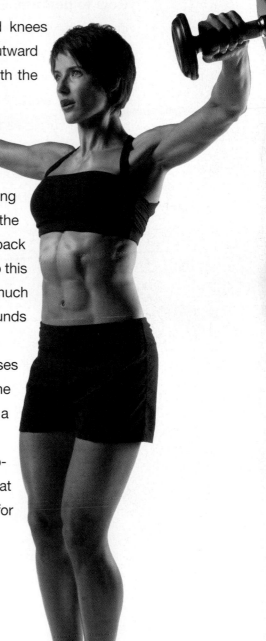

*Ab*solute Perfection

Biceps
Seated Dumbbell Curls
How to perform: Grab a pair of dumbbells and sit down on a chair. With your palms facing forward, slowly curl the dumbbells upward until your forearms are just slightly above parallel with the floor. Slowly lower the dumbbells to just short of lockout.

What they work: The dumbbell curl is another basic exercise yet to be surpassed by any fancy machinery. Besides targeting the biceps, this movement brings the forearm muscles (flexors and extensors) and brachialis into play.

Modifications: Dumbbell curls can be performed one arm at a time or simultaneously. You can also perform the exercise standing up. Just remember not to swing the body in an attempt to lift more weight.

Triceps
Dumbbell Extensions
How to perform: Sit down on a chair and hold a dumbbell over your head. With the upper arm and elbow pointing at the ceiling, lower the weight behind your head. Extend the dumbbell up until your arm is

once again locked out straight. For support you can place your free hand under the upper arm of the working side.

What they work: Dumbbell extensions primarily target the triceps.

Modifications: Some people find one-arm extensions awkward to perform so they do the two-arm version instead. In this case you grab a heavier dumbbell and hold it so your palms are facing the ceiling (as if volleying a beach ball). From here you lower the weight behind your head as before.

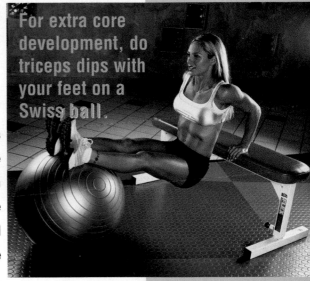

For extra core development, do triceps dips with your feet on a Swiss ball.

Chair Dips

How to perform: Place two chairs about three to four feet apart. Place your heels on one and your hands on the other. With a slight bend at the knees slowly bend the elbows and lower your body down between the two chairs to a comfortable stretch. Raise yourself upward by straightening the arms.

What they work: Chair or bench dips are a great triceps exercise. They also target the chest and front shoulders.

Modifications: As with pushups, you can change the angle by raising or lowering the level of your feet.

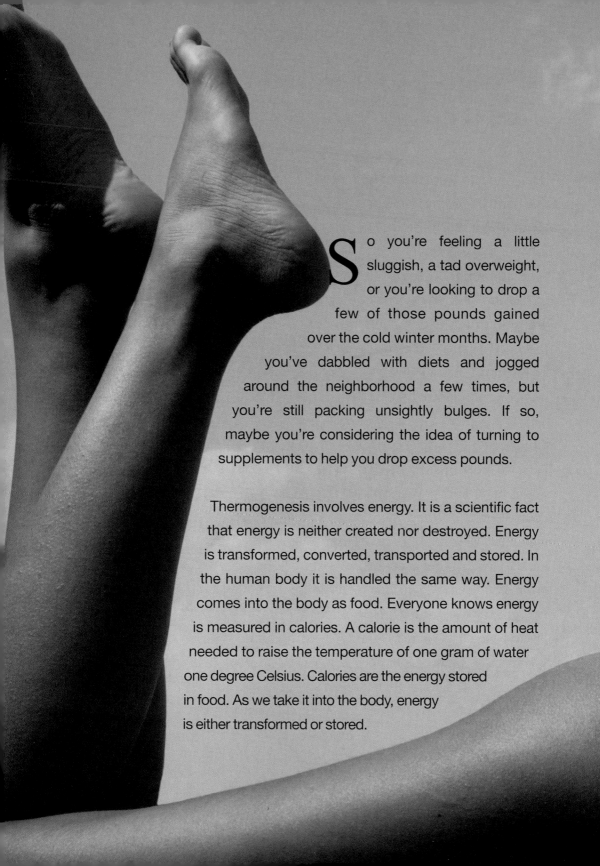

So you're feeling a little sluggish, a tad overweight, or you're looking to drop a few of those pounds gained over the cold winter months. Maybe you've dabbled with diets and jogged around the neighborhood a few times, but you're still packing unsightly bulges. If so, maybe you're considering the idea of turning to supplements to help you drop excess pounds.

Thermogenesis involves energy. It is a scientific fact that energy is neither created nor destroyed. Energy is transformed, converted, transported and stored. In the human body it is handled the same way. Energy comes into the body as food. Everyone knows energy is measured in calories. A calorie is the amount of heat needed to raise the temperature of one gram of water one degree Celsius. Calories are the energy stored in food. As we take it into the body, energy is either transformed or stored.

Chapter 8

Thermogenesis:
Turning up the Heat on Bodyfat

One of the largest energy expenditures in the human body is thermic (heat) energy. Thermic energy differentiates an endoderm – mammal, which humans are, from an ectoderm – reptile. An endoderm's basal metabolism is eight to ten times higher than that of an ectoderm. Large amounts of energy we take in are used for thermic energy. That which is not used for thermic energy is then available as net energy for the body's cellular reproduction, growth – especially in children – work muscle movement and storage. And we all know the body's unique form of storage is *fat*.

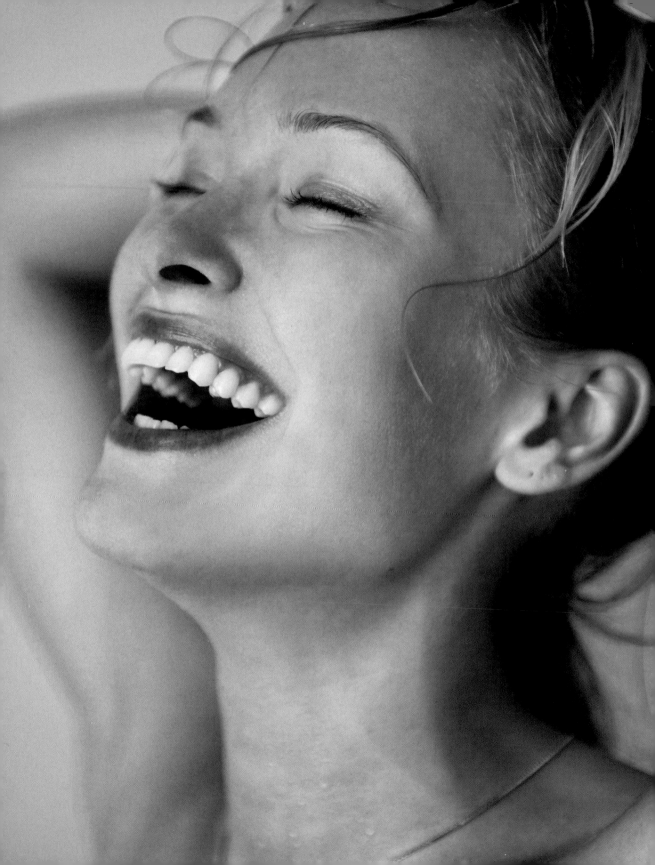

Thermogenesis means the creation of heat. There are three types of thermogenesis. The first is *work-induced,* from exercise. Muscles are forced to create heat because warm muscles work more effectively than cold muscles. The next form is called ***thermoregulatory thermogenesis.*** This function is involved with keeping the temperature of the human body regulated. The human body maintains a consistent temperature of 98.6 degrees Fahrenheit. There are two types of thermoregulatory thermogenesis: shivering and nonshivering. Shivering helps the body create heat. Muscles create the shivering. There's a tiny muscle at the end of every hair follicle that helps to create a blanket for us. Shivering heats up the body. Nonshivering thermogenesis fits into the third classification, which is called *diet-induced thermogenesis.*

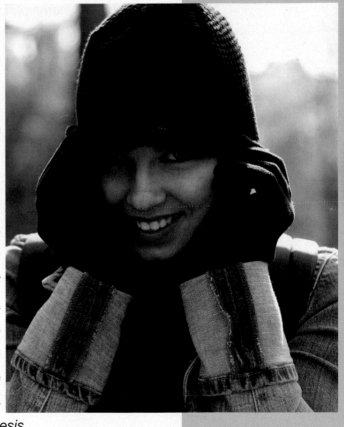

*Ab*solute Perfection

When you consume a large meal you start to get hot and sweaty. You might have to loosen your restrictive clothing. That's called diet-induced thermogenesis. It comes into play because you require more energy to digest the food you're eating. There are centers in the body capable of measuring this need and initiating nonshivering and diet-induced thermogenesis. The site most responsible for this mechanism in humans as well as other mammals is brown fat tissue. Diet-induced thermogenesis is essential for hibernating animals such as bears or small animals with a very large surface area compared to body-weight. Brown adipose tissue is also prevalent in newborn babies, who utilize tre-mendous amounts of nonshiv-ering thermogenesis to reg-ulate body temperature. As we grow older this system slows a lit-tle, but it remains hard at work.

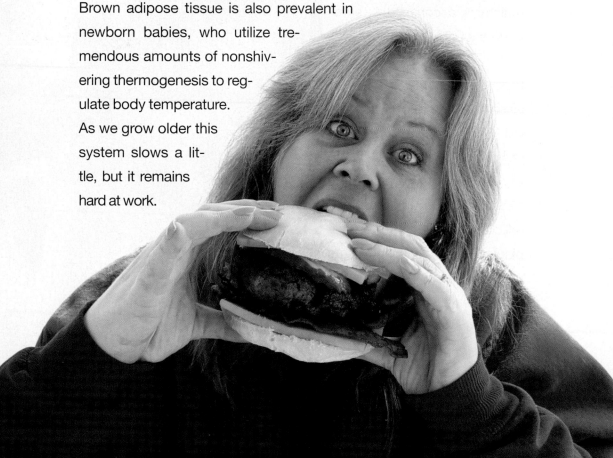

It's also important to know that brown fat (adipose tissue) is located around blood vessels and major organs. When it is triggered into activity, it causes warming of the blood and enhances blood circulation throughout the body to spread this warmth.

The thermogenic system of the body is fascinating. It is triggered by the sympathetic nervous system. Under conditions of cold or while eating a lot of food, the hypothalamus gland registers this need for energy and then triggers the sympathetic nervous system, which is an automatic nervous system. The sympathetic nervous system controls many functions, such as heartbeat and breathing, that we are not normally conscious of. The autonomic (automatic) nervous system uses energy all the time.

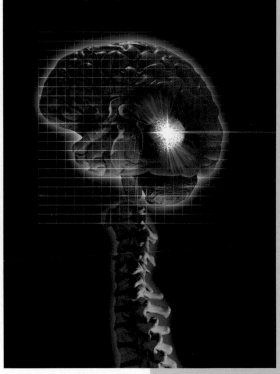

When the nervous system is triggered, norepinephrine is released and accepted by the receptors. This reaction then turns up thermogenesis. The nervous system generates other activities as well but thermogenesis is one of the most important functions involving use of energy. It is your body's thermostat. We all have a basal metabolism, which can be measured by a doctor or scientist. Your base metabolic rate tells how much energy is being consumed during the operation of your body. One of the keys to fat loss is to turn up your thermostat, or basal metabolic rate.

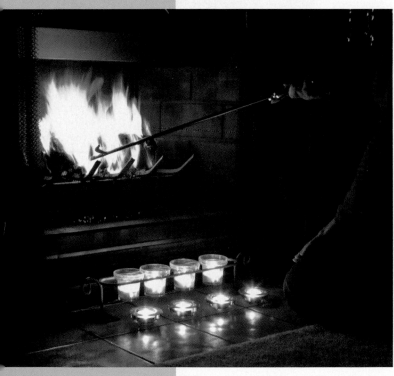

By turning up the thermostat you can cause more of the caloric energy you take in to be used for thermogenesis (as well as other areas of the sympathetic system), so that less of that intake is used for work, less is used for storage and less goes to fat. Instead the brown fat is activated, calling white blood cells into service – and that is the primary location for storage of fat in the body. Although the number of fat cells we have is consistent, the size of those cells can vary tremendously.

The brown fat cell is unique because of its mitochondria. The mitochondria are the power plants within the cells. In the brown fat cell, the unique mitochondria helps create energy. The brown fat cell is a real energy burner, burning enormous quantities of heat. Part of the problem of human obesity has very little to do with eating habits and more to do with brown-fat-cell deterioration.

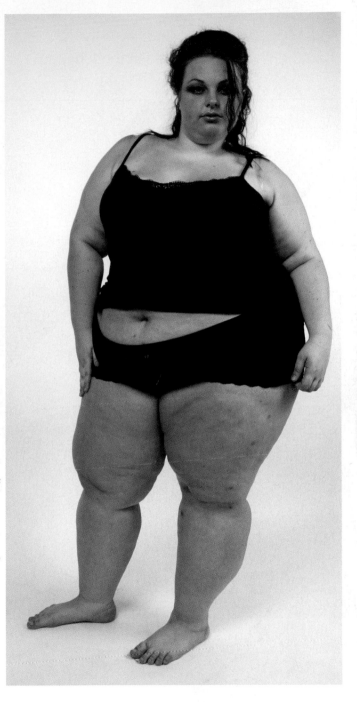

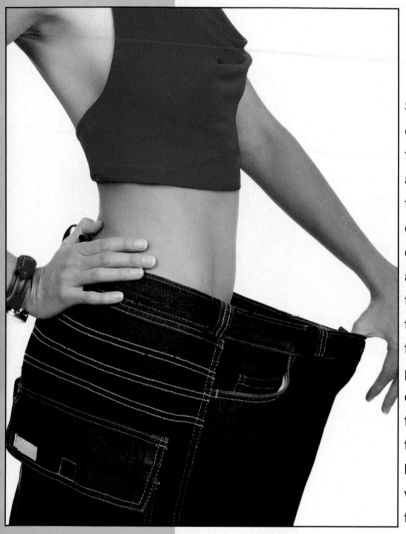

Studies about human obesity show part of the problem lies in the amount of adipose tissue activity within each of us. Some studies involving both lean and obese people have found a difference in the amount of brown fat activity. Post-obese people still have a deficiency in the brown fat system. So this system must either be rebuilt or they must always be careful about their diet.

Tricks of the Trade

Regardless of body type, the average person desires a minimum of excess bodyfat. One of the most effective "tricks" in fat-burning is ingestion of thermogenic agents. Thermogenic agents include natural plant stimulants, nutraceuticals and specific nutrients. Thermogenic nutrients can increase the number of calories you burn. Persons predisposed to obesity have a lower rate of diet-induced thermogenesis – even after they have lost weight and become lean. So for those who have a hard time losing weight, higher thermogenesis can help speed up the fat-burning process.

Some diets actually suppress thermo-genesis – the exact opposite of what you need to lose weight effectively. No wonder 95 percent of dieters fail in their efforts to lose weight!

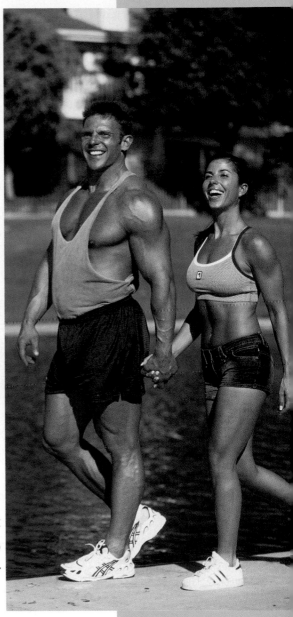

Ways to Promote Thermogenesis
- High-protein diets
- Low-calorie diets
- Low-carbohydrate diets
- Low-sodium diets

If you are having difficulty losing weight, of if you simply want to speed up fat-burning, you may want to consider using a ther-

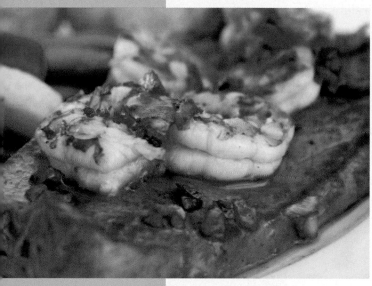

mogenic agent. The easiest way to go about starting your thermogenic program is to use safe and effective products. Choose products that contain valid thermogenic agents. They are available in the form of drinks, capsules or specialized foods. Some minerals, like potassium and magnesium, have thermogenic nesium, have thermogenic properties and can be found in thermogenic formulations.

The best time to ingest most thermogenic agents or formulations is one half hour before meals. High-glycemic meals and drinks reduce thermogenesis, and high-fat, high-glycemic meals will definitely program your body to store fat. Low-calorie diets, juice fasts, liquid fasts, and fasting in general reduce thermogenesis.

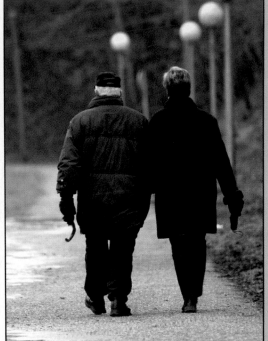

Another way to increase thermogenesis within the body is to increase your overall muscle mass. Increased muscle mass speeds the fat-burning process. You don't necessarily have to become a bodybuilder in order to increase muscle mass; even light workouts with weights can increase thermogenesis. Lower ambient temperatures (cold air) induce thermogenesis, so taking a brisk walk on a cool night and taking cool showers helps increase your metabolism for short periods of time. In addition, it has now been discovered that drinking ice-cold water increases fat burning. Drinking all your two liters of water a day at very cold temperatures could mean a 10-pound weight loss over a year, all other things being equal.

The following list will help you identify thermogenic agents known to be effective. Look for these agents on product labels, or ask your health-care professional where to shop.

129

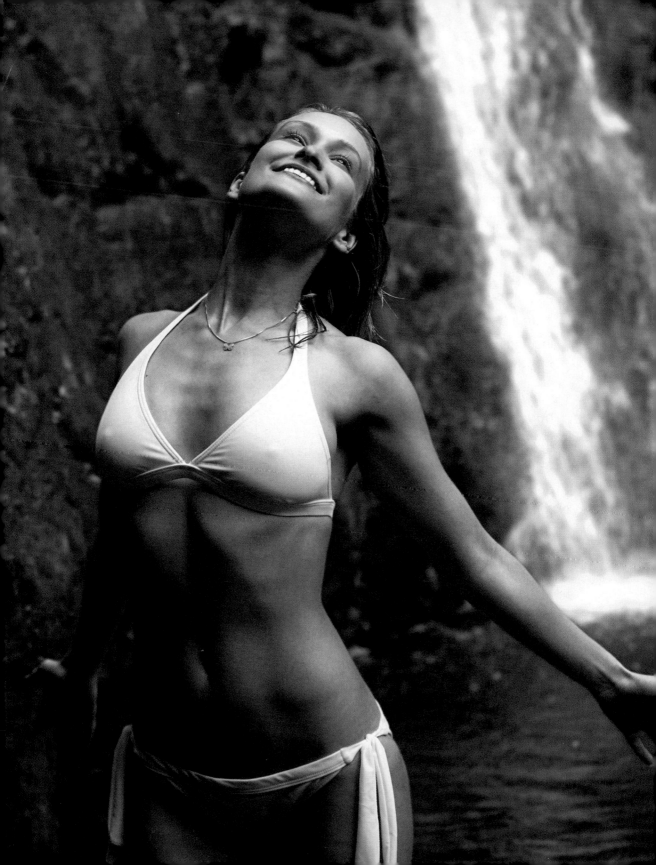

The Most Effective Thermogenic Agents

• Niacin-bound chromium (also called chromium polynicotinate)

• 5-Hydroxytryptophan, 5-HTP

• Methylxanthines (coffee, caffeine, tea, cola nut, Paullinea cupana)

• Hydroxycitrate, hydroxycitric acid, Garcinia cambogia

• Ephedrine, ma huang with caffeine (not recommended for some individuals because of the potential for increased blood pressure, increased heart rate, anxiety and insomnia, also illegal in US)

• L-carnitine

• Aspirin (1 baby aspirin with each meal. Consult your physician before using this method)

• Growth hormone

• L-arginine

Other Nutrients Acting Synergistically With Thermogenic Agents

The best time to ingest most thermogenic agents or formulations is a half hour before meals.

• Ferulic acid (found in rice bran)

• Coenzyme Q10 (frequently deficient in persons who are overweight or obese)

• Low-glycemic fruit sugars (like Ki-Sweet, which is thermogenic)

- Magnesium
- Potassium
- B-vitamins
- Niacin

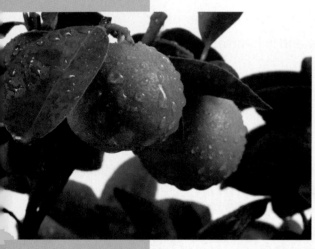

Fat-Loss Supplements in Detail
Hydroxycitric Acid – HCA
HCA is nature's fat blocker and appetite suppressor. Research over the last ten years has revealed a fat-blocking fruit acid called Garcinia cambogia. The active ingredient in Garcinia is hydroxycitric acid. HCA promotes weight loss naturally, safely and without making you feel hungry or devoid of energy.

HCA is similar to the citric acid found in oranges, grapefruit and lemons and was first identified in the late nineteenth century. However, people of Southeast Asia have used Garcinia cambogia to flavor their food and for medicinal purposes such as treating intestinal worms and other intestinal parasites for hundreds of years.

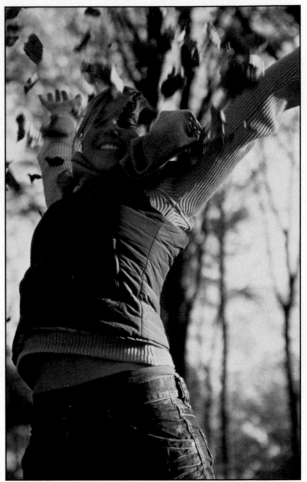

Further, Garcinia cambogia is used in many traditional recipes and is believed to aid digestion and make meals more filling. Today, people throughout Southeast Asia continue to use Garcinia cambogia in large quantities in foods and tonics.

Beginning in 1971, the pharmaceutical giant Hoffman-La Roche studied the use of HCA in treating obesity. The researchers at Hoffman-La Roche concluded that HCA blocks fat production, reduces appetite and may even stimulate thermogenesis. Better still, in all the years of its consumption, HCA has had no toxicity or adverse side effects ever reported.

HCA ignites the fat-burning engine inside your body!

In clinical studies HCA was shown to fight the most common

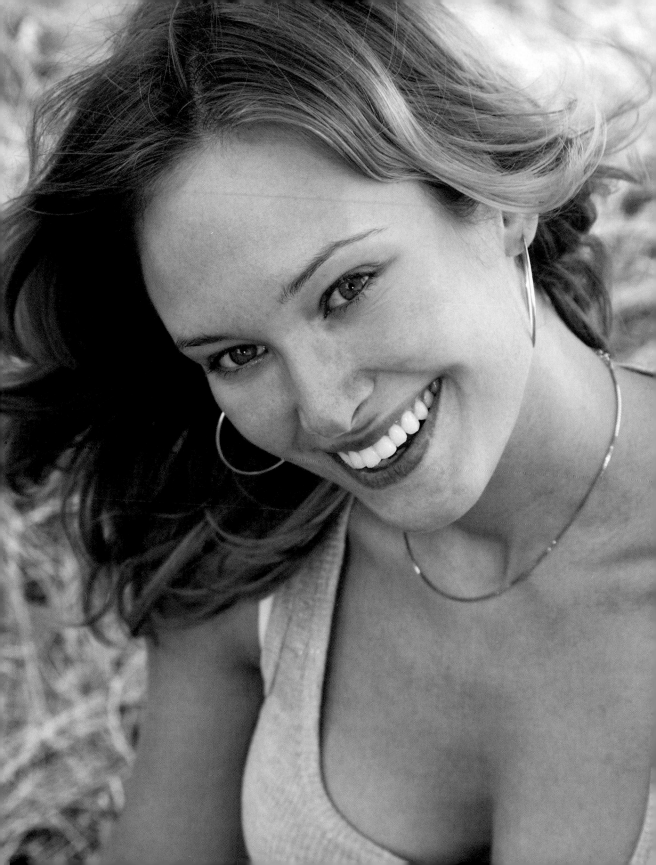

contributors to weight gain – overeating, slow metabolism and lack of energy for physical activity. Study subjects using HCA experienced a loss of bodyfat due to less food intake, increased energy and conservation of lean muscle mass. HCA is believed to promote healthy weight loss by supporting the following factors for fat loss:

Suppresses appetite – Hoffman-La Roche and Brandeis University researchers discovered that HCA sends early fullness signals to the brain through the liver, thereby reducing appetite. When appetite is reduced so is the intake of food.

Inhibits fat formation – HCA blocks the enzymes responsible for converting carbohydrates to fat. Scientists suspect that HCA produces a thermogenic effect, which may account for the ability of HCA to raise metabolism while increasing the use of stored fat for energy.

Provides extra energy – HCA diverts calories toward the production of glycogen, the special energy storage starch found in the liver and muscles, giving you more energy to get up and go.

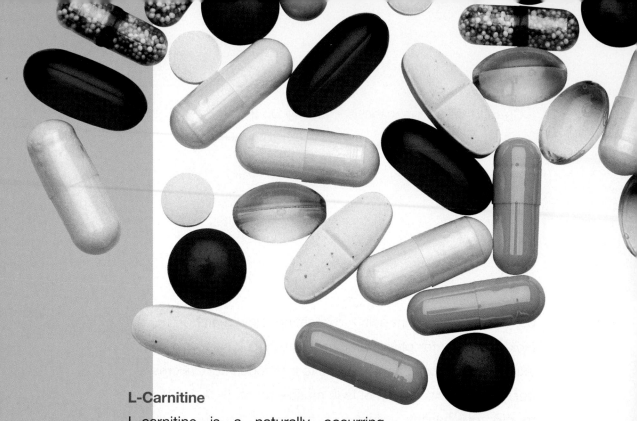

L-Carnitine

L-carnitine is a naturally occurring amino acid required for the oxidation and transport of fatty acids. Found mostly in the heart, skeletal muscle and brain, L-carnitine is synthesized in the body, primarily in the liver and kidneys, from essential amino acids obtained through the diet. Population studies have shown vegetarians are often unable to meet optimal carnitine needs. Improved lipid transport may in turn facilitate weight management, increase exercise performance and balance cholesterol levels.

L-carnitine supplementation also seems to decrease muscle fatigue by preserving muscle glycogen through the preferential use of fat as energy. L-carnitine could produce great results for decreasing weight and increasing exercise performance.

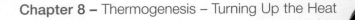

Chromium

After years of research on chromium, re-sults are for the most part equivocal in terms of fat loss, strength and muscle mass gain, some positive, some negative. The effects of chromium depend on several factors, in-cluding dosage, timing and type of chromium used. There is de-finitely an issue with chromium bioavailability, especially from food sources like brewers yeast, bro-ccoli and cinnamon. That is why supplementation with a bound form of chromium is best. This helps form stable chromium complexes.

The two most popular forms of this trace mineral are chromium picolinate, bound to a metabolite of the amino acid tryptophan and chromium polynicotinate, a special niacin-bound chromium. Although the picolinate form has been used in more studies, the polyn-icotinate form seems to be better absorbed and safer, although both forms are quite safe. At

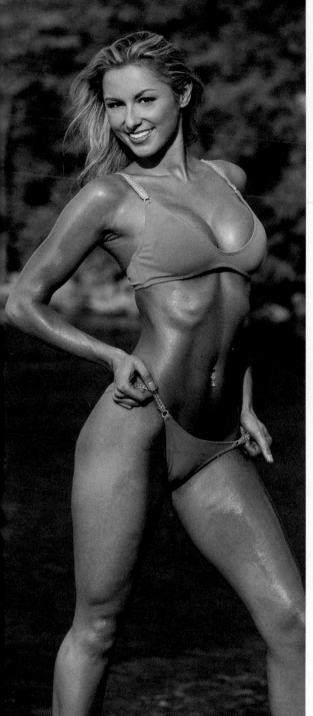

*Ab*solute Perfection

one point there was a scare about chromium picolinate damaging chromosomes and having mutagenic effects, but the studies were conducted on hamster ovary cells.

Chromium is a trace mineral of which the "Estimated Safe and Adequate Daily Dietary Intake" (ESADDI) is 50 to 200 mcg. Chromium is essential for normal protein, fat and carbohydrate metabolism. Chromium is important for energy production and also plays a key role in regulating appetite, reducing sugar craving and lowering bodyfat, according to studies. Chromium helps insulin metabolize fat. It also helps protein turn into muscle and helps convert sugar into energy. The primary function of chromium is to enhance the effects of insulin, and thereby enhance glucose, amino acid and fat metabolism. Insulin is a key hormone produced by the pancreas that helps regulate blood sugar levels, controls appetite and nutrient uptake into muscle cells.

Chromium enhances insulin sensitivity by improving insulin binding, insulin receptor numbers and insulin receptor enzymes.

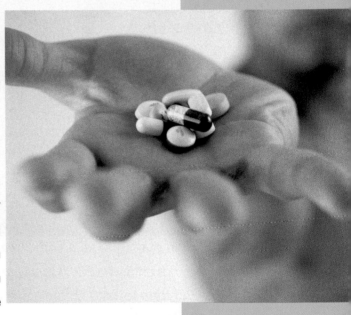

This insight may interest you: One recent study published in the *Alternative Medicine Review* stated that "the beneficial effects of chromium on serum glucose and lipids and insulin resistance occur even in the healthy." Exercise induces chromium losses in athletes and may lead to chromium deficiency resulting in impaired insulin function. Athletes may have an increased requirement for chromium. Signs of chromium deficiency include high blood glucose levels, increased cholesterol and triglycerides and decreased HDL ("good cholesterol") levels.

139

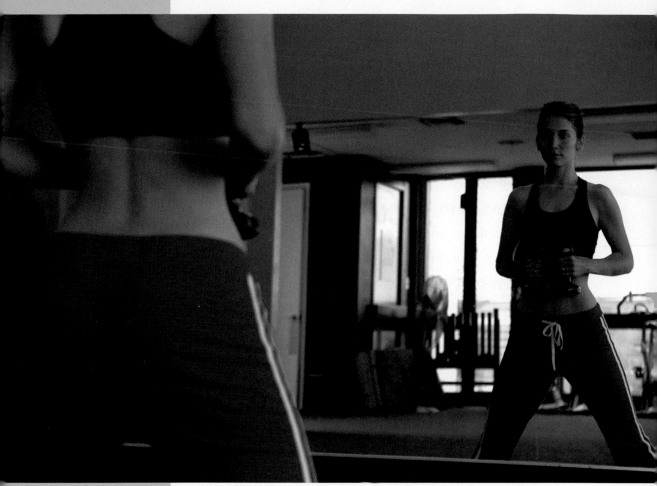

Watch out if you take chromium with iron, as they compete for absorption and binding to transferrin. It appears that it may be a good idea to take chromium and iron supplements separately. Based on research and anecdotal experience, one of the best times to take chromium is right after a weight-training workout with a postworkout shake to enhance nutrient absorption.

Vanadyl Sulfate

This form of the trace mineral vanadium is theorized to help increase glucose transport into muscle cells. It may preferentially allow for glucose to be stored in muscle cells rather than stored as fat. It is considered to be an "insulin mimic," and higher doses of substances with this property may be toxic to humans. Vanadyl sulphate also has poor bioavailability. However, it may have potential, as less toxic forms of vanadium are being discovered like bis (maltolato) oxovanadium (BMOV).

Furthermore, vanadyl sulphate has been shown to support healthy blood sugar levels in type 2 diabetics and may increase insulin sensitivity up to four weeks after vanadium supplementation has ended.

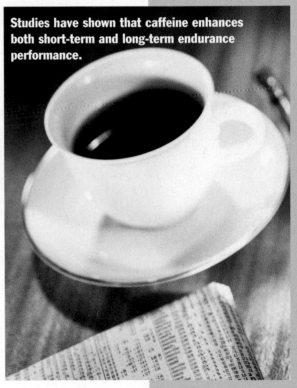

Studies have shown that caffeine enhances both short-term and long-term endurance performance.

This nutrient definitely has not lived up to its hype but still can be useful in some forms. Typical doses start at 45 mg of vanadyl sulfate taken twice daily.

Caffeine

Caffeine (chemically a methylxanthine) is one of the best, if not *the* best and most thoroughly

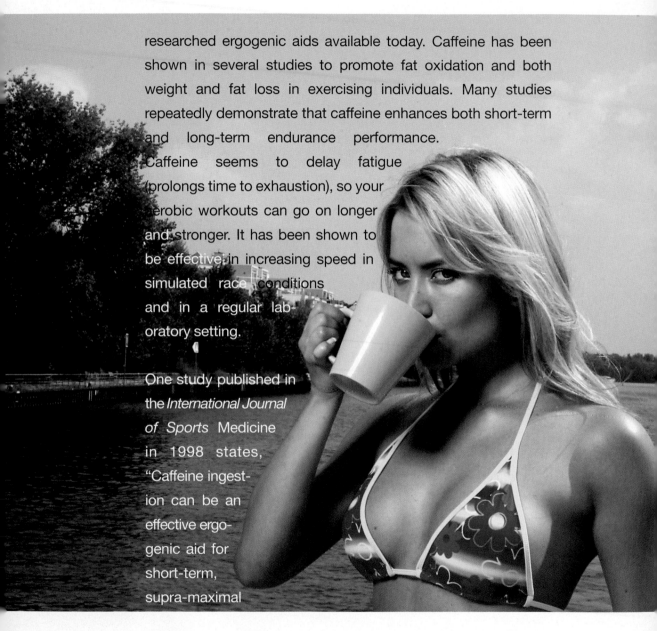

researched ergogenic aids available today. Caffeine has been shown in several studies to promote fat oxidation and both weight and fat loss in exercising individuals. Many studies repeatedly demonstrate that caffeine enhances both short-term and long-term endurance performance. Caffeine seems to delay fatigue (prolongs time to exhaustion), so your aerobic workouts can go on longer and stronger. It has been shown to be effective in increasing speed in simulated race conditions and in a regular lab- oratory setting.

One study published in the *International Journal of Sports* Medicine in 1998 states, "Caffeine ingest- ion can be an effective ergo- genic aid for short-term, supra-maximal running performance." While far fewer studies with caffeine and resistance training (weightlifting) have taken place, some evidence does suggest caffeine can increase power generated in repeated muscle contraction and enhance endurance at submaximal tension.

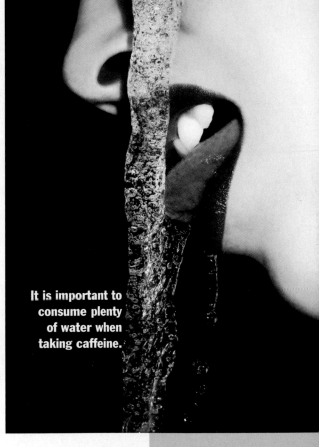

It is important to consume plenty of water when taking caffeine.

Caffeine works through several mechanisms: 1) promoting the release of stored fat to be used as energy, 2) the release of more calcium from the sarco-plasmic reticulum, thereby leading to greater muscle contraction, including greater force production by each motor unit, 3) antagonism of the adenosine receptors mainly in the central nervous system, 4) inhibition of phosphodiesterases leading to an increased level of cyclic AMP in muscle tissue, creating a more favorable intracellular environment in active muscle, 5) sparing glycogen or carbohydrate stores in muscle cells and the liver because of an increased rate of fat oxidation which could explain why caffeine delays time to exhaustion during aerobic exercise.

143

Caffeine has some diuretic properties effective in decreasing water retention in the body although it does not seem to act as a diuretic during exercise. While it's important to drink plenty of water anyway, it is especially important to consume plenty of water when taking in caffeine.

Another reaction to look out for is the effect of caffeine on blood sugar. Although the research is not conclusive, caffeine may decrease insulin sensitivity, so diabetics need to be careful. Regular consumption of high doses may also adversely affect blood pressure. *Moderation is the key.*

A good dose is 200 to 600 mg of pure caffeine about 45 minutes to one hour before exercise or a big race (levels of caffeine peak about an hour after ingestion). Taking it on an empty stomach can further enhance its effects. A regular cup of coffee has about 100 mg of caffeine per serving, but some research shows coffee is not as effective in maximizing the benefits of caffeine as is pure caffeine. The stimulation effect of caffeine usually lasts about two to four hours after ingestion, as caffeine has a short half-life in the body.

There seems to be an upper dosage threshold in terms of using caffeine as an ergogenic aid – more does not seem to be better. In fact, some research indicates taking a low to moderate amount of caffeine is equal to, if not more effective than, taking a much higher dose of caffeine. Green tea is an excellent alternative to regular coffee as it has polyphenols and a special compound called EGCG (epigallocatechin gallate), which can not only boost immune function but also enhance metabolic rate directly.

Note: Some people using higher doses of caffeine for ergogenic benefit sometimes report nervousness, jitteriness and stomach discomfort.

Citrus Aurantium (Bitter Orange)

Citrus aurantium, also called bitter orange or zhi shi is an herb containing the active ingredient synephrine. It also contains other potent compounds like octopamine and tyramine. This herb is touted as an ephedra alternative – ephedrine's calmer chemical cousin, which means it still has beta agonistic, or thermogenic/fat-burning effects, while being less stimulating to the central nervous system. Doses similar to those of ephedrine may be effective (20 mg of active synephrine after standardization per serving).

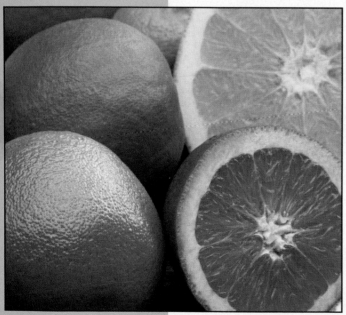

There has been a lot of research about ephedrine and caffeine combinations for fat loss, but one excellent study published in the *Current Therapeutic Research Journal* in 1999 showed a combination of Citrus aurantium extract, caffeine and St John's wort caused significant bodyfat loss in overweight healthy adults. Other research has looked at the thermogenic properties of compounds found in citrus aurantium, including synephrine and the results are promising.

EFA (Essential Fatty Acids)

EFAs can produce many benefits including;

1) improved metabolism (and therefore improved fat-losing capabilities)

2) more efficient insulin action,

3) increased growth-hormone secretion

4) improved testosterone production

5) improved blood pressure

6) liver support and protection especially with borage oil and evening primrose oil due to their GLA content

7) improved condition of hair and nails

8) improved cholesterol profile

9) decreased inflammation response

10) improved nerve function

11) enhanced immune function

12) improved energy production of cells

13) increased nitrogen retention.

There are two types of EFAs: linoleic acid and linolenic acid. Linoleic acid is included in the category known as omega-6 fatty acids, while linolenic acid – specifically, alpha-linolenic acid – is an omega-3 fatty acid. Another omega-6 fatty acid, gamma linoleic acid (GLA), is also important for good health and

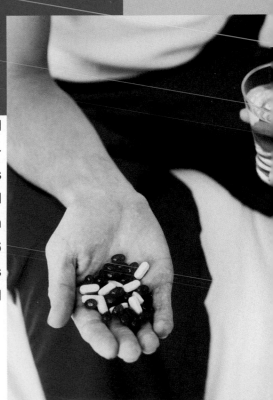

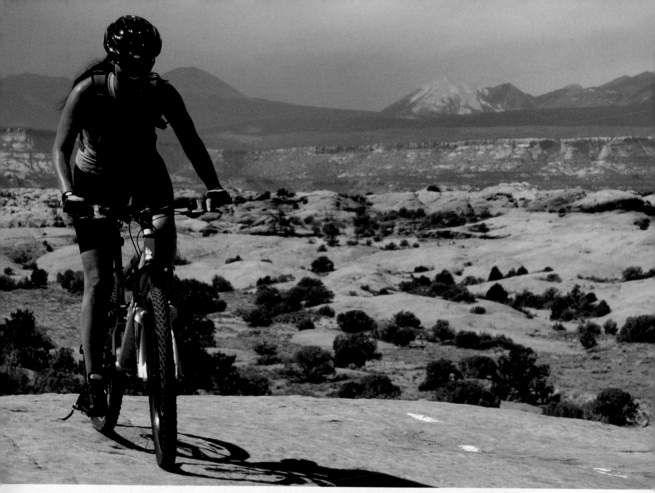

athletic performance. GLA has actually been shown to lower 5-alpha-reductase activity, which can lower the conversion of excess testosterone to DHT – a great added benefit!

There's a class of "hormone-like substances" called *prostaglandins,* which are derived from essential fatty acids. There are three classes, or series, of prostaglandins. Series 1 prostaglandins promote performance, series 2 prostaglandins disrupt performance and series 3 prostaglandins block the formation of series 2 prostaglandins. Obviously, you'd just want to use series 1 and 3.

148

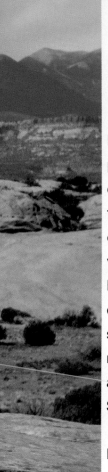

Prostaglandins can have anabolic effects in the body. Eating plenty of essential fatty acids, especially monounsaturated fats, can have a positive impact on testosterone levels. EFAs can be found in natural peanut butter, hemp seed oil, flaxseed oil, olive oil and canola oil. Eating fish, including salmon and other wild varieties, regularly provides EFAs in the diet. One study published in the *Journal of Nutrition* in 1990 showed fish oil containing EPA and DHA positively impacted testosterone synthesis. An intake of 5 to 10 grams daily of EFAs is beneficial not only for fat loss, but also as protection against heart disease and many cancers. Quality EFA products include Udo's Oil and Structured EFA from EAS.

L-Arginine

Arginine has been well researched and provides healthful benefits, especially with respect to cardiovascular health. Other research suggests it may improve exercise performance, support protein synthesis, boost growth hormone levels at higher doses and even help replenish glycogen stores postworkout. The primary mechanism of action is to boost nitric oxide production, which helps promote its many effects. Nitric oxide is basically the "signaling molecule" of muscle cells. Boosting nitric oxide in muscle tissue improves nutrient transport and blood flow. Arginine boosts nitric oxide production by stimulating nitric oxide synthase, the enzyme that makes nitric oxide. A good time

149

to take arginine is before and after a hard workout and before bedtime. Three to five grams taken at these times can be beneficial. Be careful because in some people, gram doses of arginine may cause stomach discomfort.

Momordica Charantia
(Bitter Melon Extract)

Another "insulin mimicking/blood-sugar regulating" compound with significant research behind it, Momordica charantia is actually a common vegetable with a bitter taste, hence the name bitter melon. It low-ers glucose concentration, improves glucose tolerance and promotes glucose disposal into muscle tissue. What's interesting is that even after discontinuing this nutrient for a few weeks or a period of 30 days its effects can still be seen. According to some research, it works by improving insulin secretion by beta cells of the pancreas and possibly by improving the action of insulin itself. This nutrient is especially useful to people who have late-night cravings or blood sugar imbalances. In fact, this nutrient has been extensively studied

150

in diabetics. A beneficial dose is 100 mg taken 1 to 3 times daily with meals (using a 4:1 standardized extract).

White Willow

White willow is a deciduous tree native to temperate regions of Europe and the US. White willow bark contains salicin, which the body converts into salicyclic acid. Salicyclic acid is predominantly used to decrease levels of pain. It's used for back, muscle and neck pain. In weight-loss drugs, salicin is thought to lengthen the duration of fat-loss effects of ma huang and guarana. In this respect it doesn't directly stimulate fat loss but enhances the effects of other fat-loss compounds.

You need many keys to open the door that leads to a great waistline. You must keep a clean diet, get enough cardio, and train with weights. If you are doing all these things, then a little supplementation can help, but don't expect miracles from supplementation alone.

Chapter 9

Menus, Recipes and Training Routines

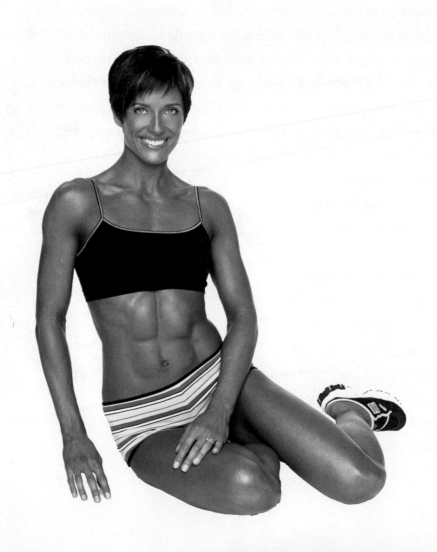

Chapter 9 – Sample Menus and Training Routines

Three Samples of Daily Menus

	Sample 1	Sample 2	Sample 3
Breakfast	Whole-wheat bagel Natural nut butter, 1 Tbls Fat-free milk, 1 cup	Oatmeal, 1 cup Fat-free milk, 1 cup Scrambled egg whites Berries, 1/2 cup	Large banana Low-fat cottage cheese, 1 cup Flaxseed, 1 Tbls
Snack	Large banana	Meal replacement bar, watch for sugar	Protein shake
Lunch	Turkey breast, 3 oz Whole-wheat bread, 2 sl Lettuce, tomato, mustard 1/4 avocado Baby carrots, 1 cup	Large green salad with diced grilled chicken breast and balsamic vinegar	Black bean and grilled veggie burrito (no cheese, no sour cream)
Snack	Plain nonfat yogurt 1 orange	Grilled veggie wrap	1 apple Small handful nuts
Dinner	Brown rice, 1 cup Shrimps, 6 oz, and Veggies, 1 1/2 cups (stir-fried with nonstick cooking spray, low- sodium soy sauce, garlic and ginger)	Pot roast, 4 oz One potato and Mixed vegetables, 2 cups, all cooked with roast.	Grilled chicken breast Baked sweet potato Grilled red bell pepper, carrots and sweet onions.
Snack	Protein shake made with 1/2 cup berries	Whole-wheat bread, 1 sl Natural nut butter, 1Tbsp Fat-free milk, 1 cup	Shredded wheat, 1 cup Fat-free milk, 1 cup

Sample Daily Calories and Fat

Breakfast:

Omelet made with four egg whites
chopped tomato,spinach
and fresh herbs
Whole-wheat toast - one slice
Natural nut butter, one tablespoon
Tea or coffee –no sugar, skim milk only

Snack:

Protein shake: Vanilla protein powder,
1 cup skim milk, 1/2 cup berries

Lunch:

Tuna salad sandwich (half-tin tuna packed in water)
on brown bread – 2 slices, no butter or margarine,
1 banana

Snack:

Caribbean-style rice and peas
Tea or coffee – no sugar, skim milk only

Dinner:

6 oz grilled chicken breast
1 large baked potato
Large helping of mixed vegetables

Snack:

1 whole piece of fruit
Nonfat yogurt

Total calories for the day = approximately 1825
Total fat for the day = approximately 22 grams

Breakfast:
2 Shredded Wheat biscuits
1 cup skim milk
1/2 cup mixed berries
Tea or coffee – no sugar, skim milk only
NB: no sugar sprinkled on cereal

Snack:
Meal-replacement bar or shake

Lunch:
Potato-tuna salad: Scoop out one cold baked
potato, mix with a half-can of tuna, 1/4 cup chickpeas,
2 Tbls fat-free dressing and 2 Tbls salsa.

Snack:
Whole -grain wrap with
Grilled chicken, lettuce, tomato
Tea or coffee – no sugar, skim milk only

Dinner:
Sliced lean beef, 4 oz, stir-fried with
broccoli, garlic and ginger
Brown rice, 1/2 cup

Snack:
1 large orange
Nonfat yogurt

Total Calories for the Day = approximately 1840
Total Fat for the Day = approximately 30 grams

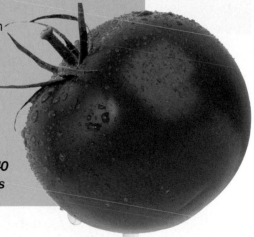

*Ab*solute Perfection

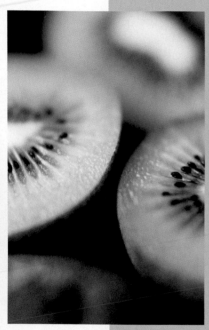

Breakfast:
1 cup oatmeal
1/2 cup sliced mixed fruit
1 cup skim milk
Tea or coffee – no sugar, skim milk only
NB: no sugar sprinkled on cereal

Snack:
2 hardboiled egg whites
2 slices whole-wheat toast
2 Tbls salsa

Lunch:
Grilled chicken breast, 4 oz
Brown rice, 1/2 cup
Mixed raw vegetables

Snack:
1 apple
1 cup low-fat cottage cheese

Dinner
6 oz fresh white fish, steamed
Oven-cooked potato "fries"
1 cup green peas

Total Calories for the Day = approximately 1800
Total Fat for the Day = approximately 22.5 grams

Menus for the Week – Monday

Breakfast	1/2 cup raisin bran cereal 4 oz skim milk 1 slice whole-wheat toast 1 Tbls natural nut butter black coffee or clear tea
Snack	1 medium banana Protein shake
Lunch	Grilled chicken breast 1 cup mixed greens salad 1 Tbsp lemon juice 1 cup skim milk
Snack	1 cup cubed honeydew melon
Dinner	1 cup whole-wheat spaghetti 1/2 cup plain low-sodium spaghetti sauce 1/2 cup cooked zucchini 3/4 cup three-bean salad 1 cup skim milk
Snack	Handful of nuts, Make sure they are unroasted and unsalted. Almonds are best.

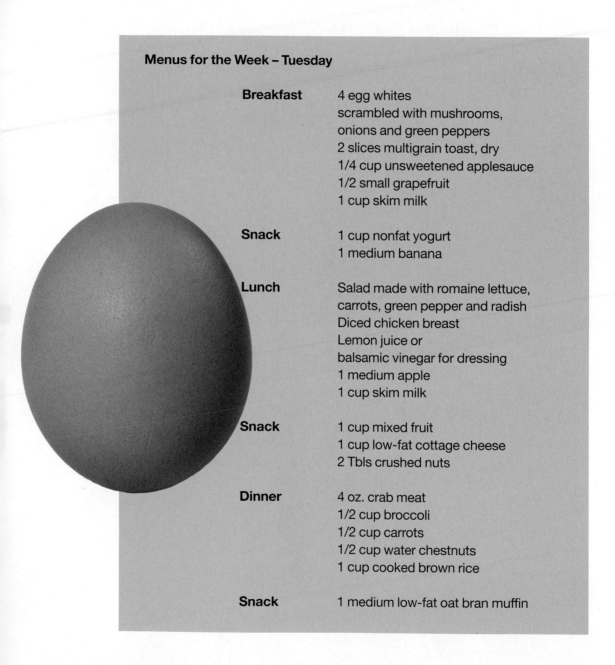

Menus for the Week – Tuesday

Breakfast
4 egg whites
scrambled with mushrooms,
onions and green peppers
2 slices multigrain toast, dry
1/4 cup unsweetened applesauce
1/2 small grapefruit
1 cup skim milk

Snack
1 cup nonfat yogurt
1 medium banana

Lunch
Salad made with romaine lettuce,
carrots, green pepper and radish
Diced chicken breast
Lemon juice or
balsamic vinegar for dressing
1 medium apple
1 cup skim milk

Snack
1 cup mixed fruit
1 cup low-fat cottage cheese
2 Tbls crushed nuts

Dinner
4 oz. crab meat
1/2 cup broccoli
1/2 cup carrots
1/2 cup water chestnuts
1 cup cooked brown rice

Snack
1 medium low-fat oat bran muffin

Menus for the Week – Wednesday

Breakfast
2 medium whole-grain pancakes
cooked with vegetable spray
1 Tbsp unsweetened applesauce
1/2 cup strawberries
1/2 cup skim milk
1 cup water, black coffee or tea

Snack
2 boiled egg whites on
1 slice whole-grain toast

Lunch
1 cup veggie and bean chili
Large salad
Lemon juice
or balsamic vinegar for dressing
1 small multigrain roll

Snack
1 fresh peach
1 cup nonfat yogurt

Dinner
4 oz. roasted skinless turkey breast
1 cup steamed mixed vegetables
1 yam or sweet potato
1 cup skim milk

Snack
handful unsalted cashews
1 apple

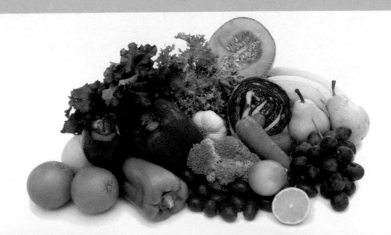

Menus for the Week – Thursday

Breakfast	1/2 cup low-fat granola cereal 1 cup plain nonfat yogurt 1 cup mixed berries
Snack	1 apple 1 slice whole-wheat bread 1 Tbls. natural nut butter
Lunch	1 cup low-sodium bean and rice soup Whole-grain wrap: 2 hardboiled egg whites with 1 tomato, diced, lettuce and sliced cucumber 10 baby carrots 1 cup skim milk
Snack	1 cup fresh fruit salad
Dinner	3 oz. skinless, baked chicken breast 1 cup mixed, steamed vegetables 1 cup brown rice 1 cup skim milk
Snack	Protein dessert shake: Chocolate protein powder with 1 cup skim milk 1 small ripe banana

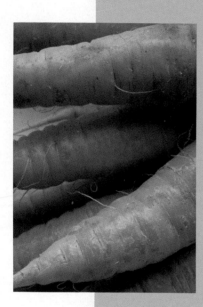

Menus for the Week – Friday

Breakfast	4 egg-white omelet made with spinach, mushrooms, onions and tomato 1 cup skim milk 2 slices of multigrain toast
Snack	10 dark grapes
Lunch	1 baked potato stuffed with 1/2 cup broccoli and 1/2 cup plain nonfat yogurt 1 cup mixed salad greens Lemon juice or balsamic vinegar for dressing
Snack	handful unsalted almonds and cashews 1 apple
Dinner	4 oz. baked salmon filet 2 cups grilled vegetables: Zucchini, onion, garlic red and yellow bell pepper 1 cup brown rice 1 cup skim milk
Snack	1/2 cup oatmeal 1/4 cup unsweetened applesauce Sprinkle cinnamon 1 cup skim milk

*Ab*solute Perfection

Menus for the Week – Saturday

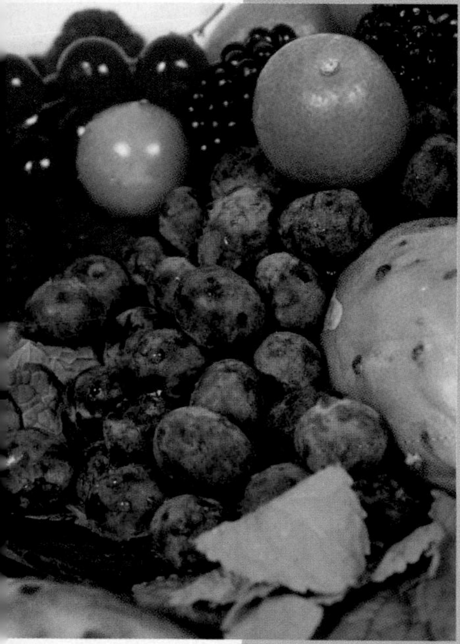

Breakfast
3 oatmeal pancakes
1/2 cup unsweetened applesauce
1/2 medium grapefruit
1 cup skim milk

Snack
1/4 cup unsalted almonds

Lunch
Whole grain wrap with
lean chicken breast and raw veggies
20 dark grapes
10 baby carrots
1 cup water
1 cup mixed fruit

Snack
2 hardboiled egg whites
1 whole grain wrap
Lettuce and tomato
1 cup skim milk

Dinner
3/4 cup spinach filled ravioli
with low-sodium tomato sauce
3/4 cup fresh green beans
1 medium oat bran roll
1 glass wine

Snack
1/2 cup unsalted cashews
1 apple
1 cup plain nonfat yogurt

Menus for the Week – Sunday

Breakfast	2 poached egg whites 1 slice whole-wheat toast 1 cup oatmeal 1/2 cup berries 1 cup skim milk
Snack	1 Banana Protein shake
Lunch	1/2 can water-packed tuna Onion, pickle, celery Lettuce and tomato as desired 1 whole grain wrap
Snack	1/2 cup low-fat cottage cheese 1 piece fruit, cut into cottage cheese 2 Tbls raisins 2 Tbls sunflower seeds
Dinner	5 oz. chicken or turkey breast 1 cup cooked brown rice 1 cup steamed broccoli 1 corn on the cob 1 whole-grain roll
Snack	1 apple Small handful unsalted nuts

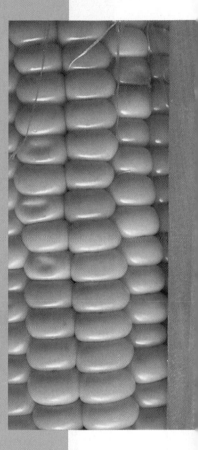

*Ab*solute Perfection

Sample Training Routine for Month 1

Monday	Tuesday	Wednesday	Thursday	Friday	Saturday	Sunday
15-20 min. Walk Ab routine	12-15 min. Stretching	15-20 min. Ab routine	12-15 min. Stretching	15-20 min. Ab routine	Rest	Rest
20-25 min. Walk Ab routine	12-15 min. Stretching	20-25 min. Ab routine	12-15 min. Stretching	20-25 min. Ab routine	10-12 min. Rope jumping	Rest
10-15 min. Jog or 30 min. Walk Ab routine	12-15 min. Stretching Weight routine	10-15 min. Jog or 30 min. Walk Ab routine	12-15 min. Stretching Weight routine	10-15 min. Jog or 30 min. Walk Ab routine	10-12 min. Rope jumping	Rest
15-20 min. Jog or 30 min. Power walk	12-15 min. Stretching Weight routine	15-20 min. Jog or 30 min. Power walk	12-15 min. Stretching Weight routine	15-20 min. Jog or 30 min. Power walk	10-12 min. Rope jumping	Rest

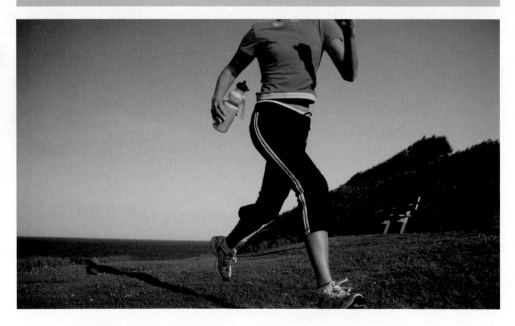

Sample Training Routine for Month 2

Monday	Tuesday	Wednesday	Thursday	Friday	Saturday	Sunday
Morning: 25-30 min. Cardio (run, power walk or swim) *Evening:* Weight routine	*Morning:* 15-20 min. Swiss-ball workout *Evening:* Ab routine Stretching	*Morning:* 25-30 min. Cardio (run, power walk or swim) *Evening:* Weight routine	*Morning:* 15-20 min. Swiss-ball workout *Evening:* Ab routine Stretching	*Morning:* 25-30 min. Cardio (run, power walk or swim) *Evening:* Weight routine	25-30 min. Cardio Ab routine	20-25 min. Jumping rope 25-30 min. Cardio
Morning: 25-30 min. cardio (run, power walk or swim) *Evening:* Weight routine	*Morning:* 15-20 min. Swiss-ball workout *Evening:* Ab routine Stretching	*Morning:* 25-30 min. cardio (run, power walk or swim) *Evening:* Weight routine	*Morning:* 15-20 min. Swiss-ball workout *Evening:* Ab routine Stretching	*Morning:* 25-30 min. cardio (run, power walk or swim) *Evening:* Weight routine	25-30 min. Cardio Ab routine	20-25 min. Jumping rope 25-30 min. Cardio
Morning: 25-30 min. cardio (run, power walk or swim) *Evening:* Weight routine	*Morning:* 15-20 min. Swiss-ball workout *Evening:* Ab routine Stretching	*Morning:* 25-30 min. cardio (run, power walk or swim) *Evening:* Weight routine	*Morning:* 15-20 min. Swiss-ball workout *Evening:* Ab routine Stretching	*Morning:* 25-30 min. cardio (run, power walk or swim) *Evening:* Weight routine	25-30 min. Cardio Ab routine	20-25 min. Jumping rope 25-30 min. cardio
Morning: 25-30 min. Cardio (run, power walk or swim) *Evening:* Weight routine	*Morning:* 20-25 min. Jumping rope *Evening:* Ab routine Stretching	*Morning:* 25-30 min. Cardio (run, power walk or swim) *Evening:* Weight routine	*Morning:* 20-25 min. Jumping rope *Evening:* Ab routine Stretching	*Morning:* 25-30 min. Cardio (run, power walk or swim) *Evening:* Weight routine	25-30 min. Cardio Ab routine	20-25 min. Swiss-ball workout 25-30 min. Cardio